SPORTS INJURIES

Self-Diagnosis and Rehabilitation
of Common Aches and Pains

Dr Malcolm Read with Paul Wade

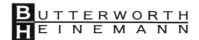

BUTTERWORTH
HEINEMANN

BUTTERWORTH-HEINEMANN

An imprint of Elsevier Limited

First published by Breslich & Foss Ltd 1984
Second edition printed in 1997
 Reprinted 1999, 2000, 2001 (twice), 2003, 2004

ISBN 0 7506 3112 0

British Library Cataloguing in Publication Data
A catalogue record for this book is available from the British Library

Library of Congress Cataloging in Publication Data
A catalog record for this book is available from the Library of Congress

Notice
Medical knowledge is constantly changing. Standard safety precautions must be followed, but as new research and clinical experience broaden our knowledge, changes in treatment and drug therapy may become necessary or appropriate. Readers are advised to check the most current product information provided by the manufacturer of each drug to be administered to verify the recommended dose, the method and duration of administration, and contraindications. It is the responsibility of the practitioner, relying on experience and knowledge of the patient, to determine dosages and the best treatment for each individual patient. Neither the Publisher nor the editors/contributor assumes any liability for any injury and/or damage to persons or property arising from this publication.

The Publisher

ELSEVIER your source for books, journals and multimedia in the health sciences

www.elsevierhealth.com

Designed by Roger Daniels
Illustrations by Tony Garrett and Don Parry
Printed and bound in Hong Kong

CONTENTS

HOW TO GET THE MOST OUT OF THIS BOOK

Top-class sportsmen and women have to be superbly fit and properly prepared, yet even they suffer sports injuries from time to time. Some are serious enough to require medical attention and specialist treatment; others are relatively minor and respond to simple home care. What many people do not realize, however, is that some injuries can be the result of poor technique rather than stress and strain. This applies to participants at all levels, from the weekend enthusiast doing jobs around the home to the international competitor.

Dr Malcolm Read, a former Olympic competitor and medical adviser to the British Olympic Association, has seen sports medicine make great advances in the last two decades, and his knowledge and experience are packed into this book.

Since most injuries can be prevented, he starts by advising you how to prepare properly. Stretching exercises for warming up and down are recommended and some sensible though simple precautions listed. An injury kit is a major essential and should always be nearby when sportsmen and women are either training or practising their sport. Some injuries are obviously serious, but you can still be of help until the arrival of a qualified person. Similarly, there are a host of bumps and bruises so common that everyone knows how to treat them – or do they? Would you bandage a blister or prick it? Read Chapter 2. Then there are the less obvious injuries – ones that hurt when you pick up a racquet or run up a hill. Locate the pain in Chapter 3, its causes and cure.

In Chapter 4, Dr Read's unique training ladders show you how to regain your general fitness; and in Chapter 5 you can find out which common technical faults cause injuries in your particular sport and how to prevent, treat or alleviate these.

This book will help you understand your injuries, get back into action afterwards and, perhaps most important, prevent problems recurring.

1

How to Avoid Injuries in the First Place

THREE SIMPLE RULES

Apart from receiving a blow or falling, the vast majority of aches and pains could be avoided if only we looked after ourselves properly. We tend to do too much too soon, such as gardening at the first glimpse of spring, or playing a sport without stretching or adequate training. With a little thought and effort, we can go a long way to prevent injuries.

1 Be fit for the task!

Even if you are generally fit, you still need to be specifically fit for the rigours of your particular task. Methodical exercise rather than violent, sudden efforts should be used to build up the correct balance of flexibility, strength and endurance. In sports, a good coaching book will set out the exercises required.

2 Warm up and warm down thoroughly!

Even if your body is not highly tuned and superfit, it will perform better when warm, just like a car engine. Warming up requires more than a few seconds flapping the arms, as the stretching exercises show. A minimum of five minutes for these and at least another five minutes to warm down, again using stretches, not only prevents stiff, sore muscles the next day, but also increases your general fitness.

3 Use the right equipment and technique!

Your body is different in shape and size from anyone else's, so the design of a running shoe or the weight of a racquet head, the position of a car seat or computer keyboard must suit you individually. Technique is just as important. If faulty, technique can even cause an injury, whether paddling a kayak or lifting a box of groceries. In sports, training a certain way may suit one person's body shape and produce a gold medal, but if those methods produce injuries in you, use other techniques that don't! Always go at your own pace.

If there is one lesson to be learned, it is that millions of injuries are caused by sudden, unaccustomed exercise or by training too hard for a sports event. These are often referred to as overuse injuries and occur when one part of the body has been asked to do too much.

Quality rather than quantity of work is what counts. More is not necessarily better! Similarly, if you have been totally inactive for years, you should allow about one month's proper training for every year of inactivity in order to regain past levels of fitness.

Think of that spring gardening session, with two or three hours spent bending, stretching and pulling. No one would dream of asking that gardener to go out and run a marathon without some preparation, yet his body is being asked to do the same sort of sudden exertion, and it does not like it!

STRETCHING EXERCISES

Whether you are a postal worker or a marathon runner, a truck driver or a tennis star, stretching exercises help to keep your muscles supple and toned for the rest of your life.

Stretching exercises can be used at any time of the day or night as part of an effort to keep fit or for warming up before training and competition. Stretching can be carried out anywhere at any time. A few moments in a lift, in between the ironing and the bedmaking, while waiting for the bus. In addition to stretching muscles, tendons and ligaments, there is evidence that proper stretching actually builds strength.

WARNING

Always relax through the tension in each exercise. Never bounce into a stretch, ease in gently. When you reach the point where you feel a pull, even a slight pain in your muscle, hold the stretch there for 10-20 seconds, breathe out and relax. Gradually you will get more and more limber. Ballistic stretching (gently swinging the leg forward and up to waist height or higher) encourages an active stretch, mimicking natural joint movements.

Throughout the book, certain exercises will be recommended as being particularly beneficial in aiding recovery. The numbers will refer to the stretching exercises illustrated below.

1

Stretches calf muscles, reducing risk of Achilles tendon tear.
With your forearms flat on a wall, keep your toes and feet together pointing straight forward.
Slowly press your hips forward while keeping your knees straight. When you feel a pull in your calves, hold for 20-30 seconds. Breathe out. Repeat at least twice.

2

Stretches calf muscle where no wall is available. This also reduces risk of Achilles tendon problems.
Keep your feet comfortably apart, your trunk upright and your upper body weight over your rear leg. Your rear foot must point straight forward. Move your front foot slowly forward. When pull is felt in the calf of your rear leg, hold for 10-20 seconds. Breathe out. Repeat at least twice. Repeat with opposite foot forward.

3

Stretches shoulder and upper back muscles. Useful for swimmers, racquet sports players, etc.

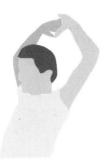

Clasp your hands behind and slightly above head height. Press shoulders and elbows back. Hold for 10-20 seconds when pull is felt. Breathe out. Repeat at least twice.

4

Stretches muscle on inside of groin. This is vital for quick side-to-side movements, and fast acceleration.

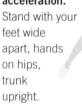

Stand with your feet wide apart, hands on hips, trunk upright.

By bending your right leg, put your weight over your straight left leg. Do not lean forward. Hold for 10-20 seconds when a pull is felt in the groin of the straight leg. Increase the stretch by leaning further over your straight leg. Keep your bottom in. Breathe out. Repeat at least twice. Repeat exercise to the other side.

5

Stretches upper back and hamstring muscles at back of thigh.

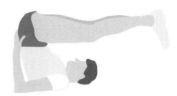

Lie on your back. Raise your legs over your head, lifting your hips off the ground. Support yourself with your hands on your hips; keep your legs together. Keep your back and legs as straight as possible. In time, your straight legs will be able to touch the ground above your head. When a pull is felt in your back and hamstrings, hold for 10-20 seconds. Breathe out. Repeat at least twice.

6

Helps side-to-side mobility.

Stand comfortably; clasp your hands at full stretch above your head. Keeping your trunk upright, lean sideways. Don't lean forward! When you feel a pull down your side, hold for 10-20 seconds. Breathe out. Repeat exercise at least twice. Repeat to the other side.

7

Helps hip and back mobility.
Stand comfortably, with your hands clasped in front of you. Slowly rotate as far as you can go to the right. Hold for 10-20 seconds. Breathe out. Repeat 5 times. Repeat exercise to other side.

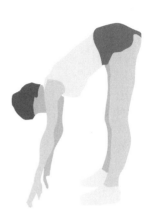

8

Stretches important quadriceps muscles on the front of your thigh.
Stand on your right leg, hold your left foot in your left hand and pull your knee back. Keep your back straight. When the pull is felt on the front of your thigh, hold for 10-20 seconds. Breathe out. Repeat at least twice. Now stretch your foot and knee as far back as you can from your bottom. Keep your knee in line with your hip to stretch both your upper thigh and outer thigh. Breathe out. Repeat at least twice. Repeat exercise on other side.

9

Stretches the injury-prone hamstring muscle at the back of the thigh.
Stand upright with your feet wide apart and your hands on hips. Push your bottom back, then pivot forward from hips, with your back straight and chest thrusting forward. Then drop your hands well in front of your feet. When the pull is felt at back of your knees, hold for 10-20 seconds. Breathe out. As flexibility increases, move your feet closer together. Repeat at least twice.

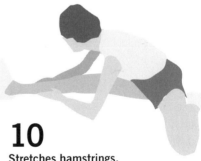

10

Stretches hamstrings, quad and adductor muscles.
Try to get your legs at right angles with your back leg bent. Then, keeping your back straight, try to place your chest over your straight leg. When a pull is felt

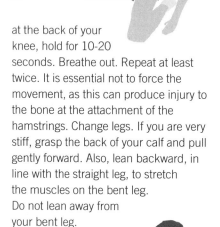

at the back of your knee, hold for 10-20 seconds. Breathe out. Repeat at least twice. It is essential not to force the movement, as this can produce injury to the bone at the attachment of the hamstrings. Change legs. If you are very stiff, grasp the back of your calf and pull gently forward. Also, lean backward, in line with the straight leg, to stretch the muscles on the bent leg. Do not lean away from your bent leg.

11

Stretches calf muscles, quad muscles and hips.
With hands on hips, move into the lunge position, with both feet pointing forward. Keep your trunk upright. Drop your weight towards your bent front leg. When a pull is felt on front of the thigh of your rear leg, hold for 10-20 seconds. Breathe out. Repeat at least twice. Repeat with opposite leg.

12

Stretches the upper end of the hamstring.
Place your right heel up on a low wall, chair, etc., preferably at hip height. Keep your back straight; try to put your chest to your knee. When a pull is felt in the buttock and behind the knee, hold for 10-20 seconds. Breathe out. Repeat at least twice. Repeat with opposite leg. Do not force this as it can produce an injury to the hamstring attachment.

SOME SENSIBLE TIPS

If we all took a few minutes every day to stretch and get fit, as many as 80 per cent of all aches, pains and injuries could be avoided. The following A-Z of sensible tips tells you how to prevent potential hazards at home or in the workplace, as well as how to prepare yourself properly for the fun and competition of sports and leisure.

Did you know that you should never train if you have flu? Or that pregnancy is no excuse for stopping exercise? Or that mouthpieces are now light, cheap and easy to wear? Read on.

Aches and pains

These are a simple indication that something is wrong. Bravely enduring pain can increase the degree of injury, so pinpoint the problem quickly, treat it properly and enjoy life more.

In the case of general aches, check your temperature and resting pulse (your pulse when you wake up in the morning, before you sit up or get up). If your temperature is up or your pulse is up by more than 5 beats per minute above normal, do not exercise.

Aeroplanes

Low cabin pressure causes feet to swell and gassy fluids to distend the stomach. Wear loose, comfortable clothes for long journeys. Air-conditioning and alcohol cause dehydration, so drink plenty of uncarbonated water.

Age

Exercise is beneficial at any age, putting off the effect of aging by giving the sense of well-being. Exercise also helps offset the effects of old age by strengthening the heart and bones, especially brittle bones (osteoporosis). But sensible precautions must be taken before engaging in a sport, especially if you are taking it up after years of relative inactivity. With age, the body's natural elasticity disappears and healing slows. It is better to do a 10-15 minute workout daily than to go all out during one session once a week. Get fit to play, don't play to get fit. Readjust your expectations, using skill and experience to replace speed and fitness.

Consult a doctor on which sport and how much activity is suitable, especially if beginning after age 50. Many take up golf or racquet games, so shoulder strength must be maintained. See: Arthritis.

AIDS

The HIV virus, which leads to AIDS, is commonly caught from unprotected sexual contacts (not using a condom). It can occasionally be caught when contaminated blood is used in a transfusion. Although the AIDS virus is easily killed by soaps and antiseptics, use rubber gloves if available when treating cuts. Anyone bleeding from a wound must be removed from playing area immediately, the bleeding stopped and the wound properly covered before the person returns to the sports arena.

Alcohol
It is not harmful in moderation. A little may calm nervous tremor, but it also decreases hand-eye coordination. Another effect is to dilate the blood vessels on the body's surface, giving a false sense of warmth while actually cooling the body faster. Therefore, a drink before going out in very cold weather can be deceptive, even dangerous. Alcohol also dehydrates. See: Aeroplanes.

Altitude and Altitude sickness
Skiers, climbers and backpackers may feel tired and breathless, and experience hammering headaches. Allow time to acclimate yourself (days or weeks depending on altitude or elevation) to less oxygen in air. The sun reflecting off snow and the wearing of heavy clothes are dehydrating, so drink more water. See: Dehydration. Altitude sickness is difficulty in breathing due to waterlogging of lungs. Move immediately at least 2,000 ft. (610 m.) lower. The effect may be lessened by acetazolamide (Thiamax).

Arthritis
There are two sorts of arthritis: degenerative arthritis caused by sheer wear and tear or aging, and disease-induced arthritis. The effects of degenerative osteoarthritis can be helped by exercises such as cycling, swimming or rowing. Avoid jarring activities, such as

running, stopping suddenly and jumping. Weightlifting exercises are possible using light weights and high repetitions. Disease-induced arthritis, such as rheumatoid and psoriatic, requires consultation with a doctor, since some conditions demand rest, while others are compatible with certain activities. See: A-Z of Medical Terms (p. 184).

Asthma
Asthmatics suffer because they cannot get enough air to their lungs. However, many world-class athletes are asthmatics. One answer is to train in a series of short sessions, with a rest in between. Swimming can be beneficial. As long as the chlorine content of the water is not too high, the damp air in indoor pools is free of pollens and other irritants. Exercise may induce wheezing (most noticeably when breathing out) in some people: This may be helped by drugs such as salbutamol (Ventolin) or sodium cromoglycate (Intal). Consult doctor. Cold weather can also spark wheezing, so use above drugs, and put a mask or scarf across nose and mouth to warm up the air you breathe. See: Drugs.

Back
Avoid or reduce backaches by improving your posture and exercising to strengthen your back and stomach muscles. See: Back (p 73).

Blood/Nosebleeds
Energetic exercise does not cause nosebleeds. If frequent, consult a doctor. See: AIDS.

Bone density

Athletic or even muscle activity helps to increase the thickness of bone. This is particularly important for women after menopause when they are prone to osteoporosis (brittle bones).

Bone growth

Stops in the mid- to late teens or early twenties. Too much exercise too early in life may result in damage to the growing points, stunting or altering the growth of the injured part.

Bowlegs/Bandy legs

Those with bowlegs may be more prone to injury, particularly in repetitive movements like long-distance running. See: Knock-knees, Pigeon-toed.

Breasts

Bouncing, unsupported breasts may be painful after exercise due to friction or torn tissue. Always wear a sports bra, which gives support without restricting movement. Blows to breast do not cause cancer, contrary to popular myth. Damaged breast fat is very tender, however, and may feel like a lump and takes time to heal. Check with doctor. See: Neck and Chest (p. 50).

Bunny hops

Leaping up and down from a crouched position is popular as a traditional exercise. However, they should be banned from training regimens. Cartilage may be torn and very few sports require this sort of leg strength in full squat position.

Calcium

See: Periods.

Check ups

A check up, including an exercise cardiogram, is essential before beginning any sport or exercise program. It will help identify any conditions or problems that may make some activities inadvisable.

Chewing gum

Inhaled chewing gum can kill. Although gum is often used by top sports stars, it should not be chewed during intense physical activity, in fun games such as tag, where sudden movements occur.

Children

Must never be sacrificed to feed ego of coach or parent. No junior champion should become a burned-out or wrecked senior. Build up stresses gradually and ensure correct techniques. Do not use age to match children, especially in contact sports. Think about matching children by size. To prevent injury, broad-based training should be used until growth spurt is over. Specific event training should be limited until this time, then gradually increased.

Clothing

Use clothing appropriate to the movements of your chosen sport. These should be comfortable rather than stylish or expensive. Jeans, for example, are too restrictive for jogging, and nylon socks do not absorb sweat. Light or reflective clothing should be worn by runners and joggers at night. See: Shoes.

Coffee

Coffee can be useful before endurance events like the marathon as it stimulates the body to release fats into the bloodstream. Muscles can therefore work longer before drawing on reserve glycogen (muscle energy source). Caffeine makes some people feel more alert, but, if taken in excess before a major competition, it can lead to a positive drug test.

Cold weather

Dress properly. The head can lose a lot of heat, so wear a hat. Protect toes, nose, fingers, and especially ears. Use lightweight waterproof suit over training clothes to reduce wind-chill effect. Cold weather may affect some sufferers of asthma. See: Asthma.

Colds

See: Head colds, Flu.

Dehydration

Often causes poor sporting performance, even in temperate climates. Increased activity means increased sweating, requiring greater fluid intake, especially when temperature is over 80°F (27°C). Whether you are an over-enthusiastic jogger or a distance event competitor (running, cycling, canoeing, etc.) you should take special care.

Check your urine colour: If it is clear, there is no dehydration; if urine is yellow, drink more water; if you are not urinating, again, drink more water, but not so much that urination is too frequent.

See: Aeroplanes, Heat/Hot weather, Salt.

Diabetes

Diabetics can take part in almost all sports after discussion and planning with doctor. Wear a medic-alert disc, a tag that identifies you as a diabetic. Usually a diabetic will require less insulin and more sugar in response to increased activity.

Diarrhoea, runner's

Many long-distance runners get diarrhoea, and even internal bleeding, sometimes showing as a black stool. It is probably due to shutdown of blood supply to intestines to divert more blood for muscles. Consult your doctor. Anti-inflammatory drugs (NSAIDs) can be a cause. Adequate fluid balance may help.

Diarrhoea, traveller's

Infection of the intestine. In tropical countries:

- Always wash hands before meals.
- Peel all fruit including grapes.
- Drink only water that is safe in approved hotels; otherwise boil it or use sterilizing tablets.
- Do not eat ice creams or swallow ice cubes from outside approved hotels.
- Beware of salads – cooked food is safer.
- Get appropriate inoculations, e.g., cholera, typhoid.
- Consult doctor about appropriate medicines.

Diet

A normal balanced diet, coupled with exercise, is essential during everyday life as well as for those in training.

Marathon runner's diet (carbohydrate loading) for more energy and less dehydration: Help load muscles with extra glycogen (muscle energy source) by training hard over 3-4 days on normal – or high-protein, low-carbohydrate diet, before training lightly for 3 days before race on high-carbohydrate, low-protein diet.

Pre-game diet: Eat 3 hours before game if possible but never less than 1-2 hours before. High-energy, quickly digested foods such as pasta, cakes and desserts are best. Low-energy, slowly digested foods like steak should be avoided. Breakfasts before morning matches should be light and continental with bread and pastries, rather than cooked, fatty foods.

Tournament diet: Games over several days deplete glycogen in muscles. Replace by going on high-carbohydrate diet, eating within 30 minutes of end of match or competition if possible.

Dieting
Cutting down on calories is the main way to lose weight. Exercise tones body muscle rather than taking off weight. Eat a sensible, well-balanced diet and exercise regularly.

Dirty clothes
Clean clothes are important. Old sweat contains germs that can cause irritating skin problems such as boils and rashes.

Double-jointed
See: Flexibility.

Drugs
Certain drugs are banned in competitive sports, even if medically prescribed. Some competitions test for traces of these in urine. Asthmatics and hay fever sufferers must check months before important competitions to see if any alteration in drugs is required to conform to rules. Even patent cough medicines, vitamins, ginseng, and other over-the-counter drugs, often contain small amounts of banned ephedrine or pseudoephedrine; they must be checked with team doctors in case they are drug positive.

Eating
See: Diet.

Epilepsy
Like diabetics, epileptics can take part in most sports. Exceptions are events where blows to head are likely, and underwater sports or climbing, where a seizure could be fatal.

Equipment
Choose equipment that suits you and feels comfortable to use. It need not be most expensive, but beware of hand-me-downs. See: Clothing, Shoes, Ski bindings.

Exposure
See: Hypothermia, Sun/Sunburn.

Eyes
Vulnerable in many sports. If protection is advised, wear it. Using protective goggles in badminton, squash or even

tennis is a sensible precaution. Swimmers usually wear goggles. Skiers and sailors need to guard against dazzling reflected light with polarized glasses. Non-glass lenses specially designed for use by sportsmen and women are available. Contact lenses help to widen field of vision.

Fatigue

This is the body's message that muscles are running out of energy and becoming choked by the body's waste products. If you persistently feel tired, however, this may be due to other causes, so check with a doctor. See: Aches and pains, Overtraining/Overuse.

Field of play

Check area of play for possible hazards, such as broken bottles, discarded cans, ice, oil. This is essential in mat areas for gymnastics or martial arts, etc., where even projecting radiators can be dangerous. Clean mats with antiseptic, especially when stained with blood.

Fitness

Are you fit to play? Hurling yourself into action after a lay-off is asking for trouble, from stiff, aching muscles to serious strains and sprains. Each activity or sport, from ballroom dancing to boxing, requires specific fitness. Check good-quality coaching manuals. Only by exercising enthusiastically at least 30 minutes every 2 days can you be fit. If you are just beginning, build up gradually: 10-15 minutes daily is better than going flat out for an hour once a week!

Flat feet

Flattening of arch between heelbone and toes, may cause strains when feet are overused. Arch support, exercises, and orthotics may help. See: Pronation/Supination.

Flexibility

Some people are congenitally hypermobile. This could mean that their knees and elbows sway back or they can put their thumb on their wrist. They do not have "double joints", only very elastic ligaments. These can be more prone to injury and even subluxing, such as when the kneecap slips partially out of place but goes back by itself.

Flexibility, lack of

This results in pulled muscles. Warm-up stretching is essential. Short muscles in particular, with no reserve in length or elasticity, may tear because of sudden slip or bend. Stretching may also contribute to muscle power, so study the stretching exercises on pages 9-12 – and then do them. Not all sports require same flexibility. Stretch for requirements of sport.

Flu

Flu is more serious than a cold. Never do energetic physical activity or train for sport with a raised temperature or with aching muscles due to fever. Flu vaccines may be given on doctor's advice. See: Aches and pains, Head colds, Resting pulse.

Genitals

These need protection in contact sports or when hard ball is used. Men should wear an athletic supporter with a hard cup even when practising for sports in which abdominal blows are common.

Ginseng

Although this herbal root is not banned by drug control rules, many so-called ginseng products may also include banned contaminants of pseudoephedrine.

Gumshields

These no longer need to be big and uncomfortable. Nowadays lightweight, translucent and cheap gumshields are available. However, even for youngsters taking part in contact sports, these should be custom-made by dentist to give a proper fit as ill-fitting gumshields could be dangerous. Properly fitted, gumshields not only protect teeth, but also help reduce likelihood of concussion in contact sports.

Hair

Keep hair out of eyes with headband. Long or loose hair could distract at a crucial moment.

Hay fever

This is an allergy to pollens, especially grass. Medications such as antihistamines and decongestants have the disadvantage of causing drowsiness. Some drugs containing pseudoephedrine may be banned in serious competitions, so check with

sports body before season begins. Equally effective drugs that are not banned are now available.

Head colds

These are caused by a virus. Antibiotics are no help, so take aspirin, (paracetamol if young child), or other painkiller; rest; plenty of fluids; nose drops (4 days maximum); throat lozenges (3 days maximum) and menthol inhalation. See: Flu, Resting pulse.

Heat/Hot weather

In hot weather, wear proper lightweight, airy clothing (cotton or cotton/mixture) and cover head and nape of neck. Under normal conditions your body needs liquids, therefore it is vital to replace fluids when exercising vigorously. In the initial stages, a single glass of water may quench your thirst, but this may not be sufficient to replace your body's lost fluids. Check the colour of your urine. The body needs 2-3 days to adjust before it tells you more fluid is needed to replace water lost by increased sweating. See: Dehydration, Sun/Sunburn.

High arches

These can cause injury since foot does not hit ground properly. However, most problems occur on top of foot, where shoe may not be cut high enough, so laces are too tight.

Hypermobile/Double-jointed

Elastic ligaments allow joints to move further than usual. The condition runs in families; hypermobile individuals may be more prone to ligament injury. See: Flexibility.

Hypothermia

Hypothermia is a dangerous chilling of the body. It often occurs in water-related sports like canoeing. Hypothermia is described as the "number-one killer of outdoor recreationists" by the U.S. Forest Service, which defines it as the "rapid, progressive mental and physical collapse accompanying the chilling of the inner core of the human body… cause by exposure to cold, aggravated by wet, wind and exhaustion". A waterproof outer layer of clothing helps retain body heat. It is not enough merely to protect the upper body. For hiking, waterproof trousers as well as anoraks are advised as wet legs can lose large amounts of heat. Get anyone who has fallen in water out as soon as possible. If help is not available, remain still in water to conserve heat as swimming warms limbs but cools core temperature. Hypothermia victims are irrational, have slow responses and speech and vision difficulties and are cold to touch. Their pulse and breathing are weak.

Recovery: Remove their wet clothes and warm gradually in a sleeping bag, or between two bodies. Hikers and mountaineers should carry space blanket or large plastic bags for this eventuality as wind and wetness chill fastest of all. Application of sudden intense heat is dangerous. Seek medical help immediately.

Indigestion

This pain in the pit of the stomach is often due to tension. Antacids give relief, anti-inflammatory drugs make it worse. Some sports, like cycling, encourage heartburn and stomach gas to press under diaphragm. Use antacids and peppermint to bring up wind before competition and avoid carbonated drinks. One teaspoon of bicarbonate of soda (baking soda) in a cup of water is a simple antacid.

Influenza

See: Flu.

Jet lag

Your body needs 24 hours per hour of time change to adjust fully. Therefore, fatigue may be felt even when sightseeing or exercising normally during first few days of adjustment. Prepare ahead of time by eating and sleeping on the destination's time clock. Some may find that sleeping tablets help this adjustment; consult your doctor. See: Aeroplanes.

Jewellery

It should never be worn for sporting activity, especially pendant necklaces, earrings, finger rings or watches as they can cause injury to wearer or opponent.

Kit, injury

Even the occasional sportsman or woman should have an injury kit handy. See: Your Injury Kit p. 26.

Knock-knees

They can put extra strain on knees. Corrective orthotics in shoe may help; consult orthopedist. See: Bowlegs/Bandy legs, Pigeon-toed.

Legs of unequal length

Non-sports doctors feel this has little effect unless difference is at least 1 in. (2 cm.). However, runners may suffer from leg strain and back pain. Raising the heel or using an extra innersole will help shorter leg. Note that when osteopaths use the expression "short leg", it refers to a twist of the pelvis, not the length of your leg.

Liniment

It smells sporty, but its warm sensation has no deep-down effect on muscles and is no substitute for a proper warm-up.

Menstruation

See: Periods.

Nails, finger and toe

Nails should be trimmed frequently. Toenails should be cut square to avoid ingrowing. Fingernails should be short and neat, especially for catching sports.

Nosebleeds

See: Blood/Nosebleeds.

Orthotics

See: Pronation/Supination, Flat feet.

Overtraining/Fatigue

If overtraining causes fatigue, 3 weeks total rest should help.

Overtraining/Overuse

Overuse is a common cause of injury in non-contact sports. Do not work through pain. Instead, build up the body to withstand workload. Training schedules must be individual, to suit a specific body. A rest day should be built into training week.

Overweight

Athletic activity can help reduce weight if planned in conjunction with specific diet and training. A heavy build puts more strain on lower legs so be careful when choosing footwear. If taking up a sport after years of inactivity, have a medical checkup and ease gently into action. Body fat measurement is a better indicator than weight measurement as fat is replaced by muscle when exercise is combined with a planned diet. Therefore an increase in weight might not reflect a gain of fat but rather in muscle.

Periods

There is no reason why women with normal periods cannot compete. World and Olympic titles have been won at all stages of monthly cycle. Painful periods with premenstrual fluid retention can be eased. Consult doctor. Very light or absent periods may be related to training and not disease. Young gymnasts, for example, may experience delay in the onset of periods; this is not a problem. Long-distance runners may stop having periods. Again, this is not a problem in itself, but bone density may be diminished, leading to stress fractures.

Calcium supplements should be taken. To rest/reduce jarring the bones, training should include non-running endurance exercises such as cycling. See: Pill, the.

Physical handicap

The inspiration for the Special Olympics was the Stoke Mandeville Games for the physically handicapped, initiated by Sir Ludwig Guttman in 1952. His theory was that sports and exercise would both regenerate muscle and provide mental stimulus to help even the seriously handicapped to survive. This has gained international acceptance, and the Special Olympics are now having to reassess handicap categories to cope with increased demand and to ensure fairness of competition.

Pigeon-toed

This term describes feet that turn inward, so toes on one foot point at toes on other. Most problems occur from overuse. In long-distance running, pigeon-toes can affect feet, legs, knees and hips. See: Bowlegs/Bandy legs; Knock-knees.

Pill, the

This is often used by top-class women competitors to control painful periods and/or regulate menstrual cycles. On medical advice, periods may be postponed by carrying on with following month's supply (or even for few extra days) of pills without the normal seven-day break, then resuming dosage as normal. This should be planned and carried out several months before an important event.

Pregnancy

If active before pregnancy, women can continue sports with no ill effects as long as they feel comfortable. Baby is well protected in bag of fluid. However, stop exercise immediately if spotting blood or low stomach or back pain occur. Consult doctor.

Pronation/Supination

When running, the way the foot lands is important. First of all, the foot strikes the ground firmly, rolling outward in what is called supination. The foot then rolls in to adapt to the contours of the ground; this is called pronation. The foot then stiffens again as it pushes off from the ground – supination again. Too much pronation can cause foot, leg, knee, hip, back troubles; specially designed inserts for the running shoe, called orthotics, may help. They need expert fitting to be most effective.

Pulse rate

A fit person will do the same amount of exercise at a slower heart rate than a less fit person, who will draw on more reserves for extra work. Stamina, or aerobic, training makes heart stronger and lungs more efficient. Normal heart cannot be damaged by exercise. See: Resting pulse.

Resting pulse

This is the pulse taken when first awake and before getting up. Aerobic fitness lowers resting pulse. An elevation of this pulse rate by 5-10 beats per minute indicates that you should not train.

Salt

Salt is lost from the body in sweat and must be replaced by adding it to food and drinks or even by taking salt tablets. But the most vital replacement is liquid. Special drinks containing salt and other chemicals lost in sweat may also have sugar for energy. See: Dehydration.

Senior citizens

See: Age, Arthritis.

Sex

By all accounts, sex is better when both partners are fit and healthy. Even professional sportsmen and women feel no need to abstain before competition. If anything, relaxation after lovemaking calms pre-game tension. However, recent research suggests that the aggressive, competitive instinct may be blunted by precompetition sex. See: AIDS.

Shoes

Sports shoes have a low broad sole for change-of-direction games and thick, shock-absorbing soles for running. Check shoes regularly by standing them on a table and looking at them from behind. If shoes lean in or out, then the heel cup/uppers may be broken. This often occurs before the sole wears out, but shoes still need replacing. Beware of high stiff Achilles heel tags, as these may cause injury. When buying shoes, check whether they are competition shoes, trainers or merely for leisure wear. Some shoes are designed to help pronation or supination.
See: Pronation/Supination.

Ski bindings

These should be checked before skiing each year. They need to be freed up each morning during skiing, as overnight cold stiffens moving parts.

Smoking

A drop of nicotine on an artery contracts it, allowing less blood through. This causes high blood pressure and means less blood gets to muscles. Smoke clogs fine filters of lungs and various chemicals displace oxygen in red blood cells. Smoking is also known to cause cancer.

Socks

When worn for soccer, basketball, etc., should be kept up by broad tape (not string, which could cut off circulation). Holes can cause blisters. See: Clothing.

Sun/Sunburn

Apart from the face, the top of a bald head, back of neck, nose, shoulders, tops of ears, feet and knees are especially vulnerable to sunburn. Build up exposure slowly. Sunscreens are effective. Water and snow may double sun's effect by reflection, while swimming cools down the body's warning sense of discomfort or heat. Use moisturizing creams after exposure. Continual exposure increases chance of skin cancer, which is why many top athletes who perform for long periods in the sun wear brightly-coloured protective creams. Prevention is better than cure, but for serious sunburn, consult doctor. See: Dehydration.

Sweatbands

These help keep sweat and long hair out of eyes, but should not be so tight as to restrict blood supply to scalp. Sometimes a smear of petroleum jelly over eyebrows helps sweat run away from eyes. Wristbands prevent sweat running onto grip (for racquet games).

Teeth

Regular dental checks will prevent a sudden abscess from ruining competition or recreation.
See: Gumshields.

Temperature, raised

If this occurs, stop all training. No sporting injury (apart from dehydration) makes your temperature rise. Resume training only when feeling completely well again, with temperature and resting pulse back to normal.

Tetanus

Sports people should have regular protective injections. Consult doctor.

Urine, blood in

This needs to be checked by a doctor. It may be result of physical activity, such as a long-distance run. Some individuals break down muscle tissue during heavy exercise and produce red urine (myoglobin or haemoglobin). This is not dangerous.

Varicose veins

Exercise generally improves deep veins. Elastic supports can be worn.

RICE

RICE is the simplest and most efficient remedy for a host of injuries, and yet many sportsmen and women disregard this valuable aid.

DO NOT IGNORE THIS ADVICE

The combination of **R** (rest), **I** (ice), **C** (Compression) and **E** (Elevation) helps to reduce swelling and restrict the spread of bruising, both of which can slow down the healing process. As soon as possible after sustaining injury, you should apply ice and bandages and raise the injured part. At the same time you can enjoy the post-game socializing, happy in the knowledge that you are doing something positive to heal your injury.

REST

Do not work through the pain. Rest the injury as soon as possible. The first 6 hours are the most vital. Most injuries require 48 hours rest before mobilization should start. If you try to move the injured part too soon, the scar tissue tends to thicken.

ICE

Apply ice pack (or cold water if ice not available) to injured area for 5-10 minutes every hour, if possible, over 48 hours (not in bed, at night, of course). This reduces bleeding from torn blood vessels.

WARNING

Ice may be colder than 32°F and must not be put directly onto skin as this will cause an ice burn. Wrap the ice in a cloth, tea towel, etc. It may cause nerve damage if left on too long (neuropraxia).

COMPRESSION

To control swelling, bandage injured area firmly, but not so tightly that it is uncomfortable. Always be prepared to adjust tightness as necessary. Combined ice/compression kits are available from specialty sports shops and pharmacies, as are chemical coolants.

ELEVATION

Allow blood to flow towards heart by raising injured area, even if you are in the office. Rest a leg on a chair, for example. This reduces pressure of fluid on injured area.

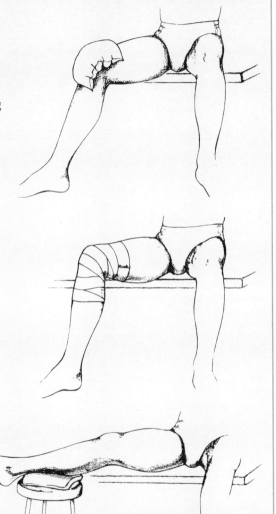

YOUR INJURY KIT

If there is one essential standby in the home and workplace, or for the sportsman or woman, it has to be the injury kit. Think ahead: don't ruin your day for lack of something as simple as a plaster. There are first-aid kits on the market, but it's just as easy (and cheaper!) to assemble your own. Stage 1 is our recommended minimum, but the more sports you or your family participate in and the better you are at it, the more you need to be prepared. Add stage 2, then 3 – and even 4 for team events.

STAGE 1	STAGE 2	STAGE 3	STAGE 4
Home	**Workplace**	**Recreation**	**Serious sports**
Box of different-	Safety pins	Strapping tape and/	**events**
sized plasters	Sling	or brace	(for use by qualified
Sterile gauze pads	Scissors with 2 in.	Underwrap	medical staff)
(clean, ironed	(5 cm.) blades, for	Tincture of benzoin	Fracture boards or
handkerchief will	medical use	compound to stop	blow-up splints
do) 4 x 4 in.	Needle	tape hurting skin	Scoop stretcher
(10 x 10 cm.)	Cotton wool	Aerosol coolant	Oxygen and mask,
Gauze bandages	Antiseptic	spray	ambu bag
Box of bandages of	fluid/wipes	Plastic or "second	Suture kit
various sizes	Tweezers	skin" product for	Embucrylate
Plastic bags for ice	Rubber bands	blisters	Cervical collar
(or package of	NSAIDs or non-	Fluid replacement	Emergency
frozen peas –	aspirin painkiller	drink	resuscitation
ideal shape for	Adhesive tape	Nail clippers	equipment
applying to	Portable razor	Petroleum jelly	Defibrillator
injuries) or ice	Butterfly bandage or	Baby oil/	Emergency drug
pack kept in	adhesive plaster	oil of wintergreen/	cupboard
freezer	sutures	massage cream	(checked by
Scissors, for general	Eyebath and	Orthopedic felt for	doctor to ensure
use	eyewash	padding	present and up to
This book and first-	Thermometer	Elastic knee/ankle/	date)
aid book	Antacid tablets	elbow support	
		Foot powder	
		Anti-inflammatory	
		drugs (NSAIDs)	

Too often friends will borrow the scissors or use the last plaster without replacing it, so post a list of contents on the outside of your bag and check regularly. Make sure the telephone number of your ambulance service, doctor or sports injury expert is written or taped on it. This should be checked and updated regularly.

2

Guide to Treatments

A-Z OF SELF AND MEDICAL TREATMENTS

The A-Z of treatments – both self and medically prescribed – tells you what some of the more commonly used forms of treatment for injuries actually do to help you. These can apply whether you have fallen off a ladder while painting your kitchen or taken a tumble when cycling. It is followed by a list of common ailments or minor injuries and advice on how to cope with them.

Acupuncture
Oriental system of inserting needles into specific parts of the body to raise the pain threshold.

Adverse neural tension
A technique for treating trapped nerves from disc etc.

Amino acids
Protein building blocks of body. Claims for amino acid supplements may be exaggerated, but "branched-chain" amino acids may help fatigue. Tryptophan known to have produced bad reactions.

Antibiotics
Chemicals that kill off bacteria that cause infections. Are ineffective against viruses such as flu or common cold.

Anti-inflammatory drugs/NSAIDs
Neutralize inflammation produced by damage to body. Known as NSAIDs (non-steroidal anti-inflammatory drugs). Also available as gel or cream. Aspirin is best known, but there are many others on the market. Must be taken with food as they can cause indigestion and even stomach ulcers. Some people have an allergic reaction to these drugs. Consult doctor.

Aspiration
See: Draining with needle.

Aspirin
Excellent anti-inflammatory agent (see above). Standard dose is 2 tablets with each meal at minimum 4-hour intervals; also before going to bed with, say, glass of milk. Continue for 48 hours. Paracetamol is recommended for children under 10.

Beta agonist
Treatment for asthma
See: Salbutamol.

Beta antagonist/Beta blocker
Calms nervous tremors, may cause asthma but in several sports is banned by authorities. Used for raised blood pressure or angina. Can reduce exercise performance. See: Calcium antagonist.

Bone scan
For diagnosis of stress fractures. Uses injection of Technetium, a radio-active substance that is the approximate equivalent of 1 x-ray.

Braces
Used to support joints, these are more and more "high-tech", often made of

strong, lightweight materials. Although knee braces are unlikely to prevent injury to an undamaged joint, their pressure on the skin may enhance awareness of joint position and improve overall control. Some sports do not permit braces that could inflict injury on opponents, while some coaches require their players to use joint protection for areas such as the ankle.

Calcium antagonist
Drug for angina and blood pressure. Allowed in sports where beta blocker banned; more efficient than beta blocker if exercising.

Compress
Firm bandaging that may also hold hot or cold pad onto damaged area.

Cortisone injection
Reduces inflammation. Cortisone is a very useful drug, but overuse may lead to problems. The injury may be more painful for 48 hours after injection. Banned by sports organizations if taken by mouth or injected for general (systemic) rather than local use, such as asthma. Special dispensation may be obtained with prior appeal to the sports organization.

CT scan
Type of body scan using computerized tomography. Excellent for bones; good for discs, brain and soft tissues.

Draining with needle
Releasing fluid from injured area. Also called aspirations.

Echocardiogram
Ultrasound screen of the heart to monitor blood flow, valves and thickness of heart wall.

Effluage
Massage technique that works damaged cells and fluid away from injury toward heart.

EKG/ECG (Electrocardiogram)
An EKG/ECG is an electrical trace of heart muscle activity, looking for abnormalities.

Enzyme cream
Contains chemical to increase blood supply and "digest" bruise.

Epidural injection
Spinal injection, commonly used for women giving birth, that temporarily numbs and paralyses lower limbs and pelvic area. It is also treatment for sciatic pain. May be given by translumbar (between the vertebrae) or caudal route (with hole near the tail of the spine). May be given to out-patients in dilute form for sciatica (nerve pain in legs) as no temporary paralysis of lower legs results from this treatment.

Erythropoietin
Hormone to stimulate production of more blood cells. Illegal in sports use.

Faradism, differential
A machine that causes muscles to contract by applying an asymmetrical alternating current of electricity.

Heel raise
Rubber insertion in shoes to alter angle
of foot as it strikes ground when walking
or running. Can also help early treatment
of Achilles tendon problem.

Ice
Alternatives are cold water; cooling gel;
chemical freezer; a bag of frozen peas;
anything that cools painful area.

ICE
Ice, Compression, Elevation. See: RICE.

Injections
In this book, the term refers to those
made directly at the seat of injury.

Interferential
Electromagnetic wave that penetrates
deep into body tissue. Stimulates muscle
contraction and to reduce level of pain.

Ladders
The author's rehabilitation plans. See
Chapter 4.

Laser
There are two kinds of laser:
Surgical: Used as an accurate cutting
instrument in surgery.
Therapeutic: This non-cutting laser
increases the rate of healing. Most
beneficial for 3-4 treatments; less
effective after that.

Manipulation, self, surgical
Technique of locking some joints so that
others may be freed.

Massage
Designed to warm up muscles and skin
and to help clear fluid and bruising,
depending on technique used.
Cross-frictional: Rubs skin across muscle
and tendons rather than along their
length.
Deep friction: Uses firm pressure to get
at deeper tissues.

Menthol crystals, inhalation of
Clears sinus and nasal passages. Only
requires about two crystals dissolved in
hot water. Cheap, easy to obtain and not
drug positive.

Mobilization
Moving joint or muscle through its
normal range.

MRI
Magnetic Resonance Imaging. A body
scan for bone, disc, brain and soft tissue.

Muscle relaxant
Drug that reduces tension or excitability
of a muscle. May be mild or major, as
used in surgery. Some types, such as
beta blocker, banned in some sports.
Check with medical adviser.

Nose drops
Reduce swelling in nasal passages,
improving airflow. If used more than 4
days, however, may perpetuate nasal
problem.

NSAIDs/Anti-inflammatory drugs
Non-steroidal anti-inflammatory drugs,
the best known of which is aspirin.

Orthotics

Various devices made to fit in shoe, aimed at correcting or altering foot position to help overuse strains of foot, ankle, knee or back. They range from heel and arch inserts to expensive, custom-made insoles. They are useful, but not cure-all.

Painkillers

May work to stop brain from telling you something hurts or may calm painful area, e.g., morphine, aspirin.

Physiotherapy

Includes massage, heating and mobilization treatments.

Plaster cast

Plaster of Paris cast that prevents movement of joints or broken bones. Lightweight fibreglass may also be used.

RICE

Rest, Ice, Compression, Elevation – the most underrated but effective way of dealing with injuries (sometimes referred to merely as ICE). See: RICE (p. 24-5).

Salbutamol

A beta agonist to help asthma.

Shortwave diathermy

Injury treatment using a pulsed electromagnetic instrument.

SPECT scan

A highly sensitive body scan. See: Bone scan.

Sling

Triangular bandage tied around neck to support weight of forearm and elbow.
Collar and cuff sling supports injury from wrist to neck.

Splint

Solid object to which damaged part may be strapped. Prevents painful movement of joint or fracture.

Steristrip/Butterfly plaster

An adhesive plaster designed to pull two sides of a cut together.

Strapping

Used to support muscle or joint, giving added strength. May be stretch elastic or non-stretch adhesive tape. (See diagram, p. 113.)

Sugar injection

Contains dextrose sugar; used to promote growth and strength of back ligaments.

Support corset

Strap-on corset that may have strengthening bones (plastic or metal). Used to support back. Physical reminder of correct back position when gardening, lifting, etc.

Sutures

Stitches of catgut, nylon or silk for repairing cuts or surgery.

Taping joints

May strengthen injured part, particularly ligaments surrounding joint. Stops relevant bones from stretching too far apart. Once ligament is pain free, continue taping or use elastic support for a further 6 weeks so full strength is regained. Then (there are two schools of thought) either: (a) strap joint for activity, thus preventing damage and keeping joint stable but spreading torque or load onto other joints; or (b) stop strapping, so that torque may be shared by this joint as well as others. This last theory says that the immobile or stable joint can't take its share of load and so overloads others. Custom-made lace-up ankle supports, elastic knee, elbow, wrist supports may be as effective. See: Braces.

Self-taping
Consult physiotherapist or experienced adviser if possible. Shave hair or apply tincture of benzoin compound or thin rubber underwrap to stop strapping burns. See: Braces.

TENS
Stands for Transcutaneous Electrical Nerve Stimulation. Way to stop pain without using drugs. May stimulate muscle contractions.

Traction
Pulling apart from both ends (broken bones, spinal disc) to allow damaged parts to return to normal position.

Ultrasound
High-frequency sound wave that vibrates and loosens scar tissue, also produces heat at deeper level; can be used to scan muscles, tendons and body organs. Can increase rate of healing.

Warm baths
Increase blood flow and warm joints. Damaged joints may then be moved more easily.

Water tablets/Diuretics
Make you urinate more frequently. Often taken by people with damaged hearts so that amount of fluid in circulation is less; may ease premenstrual breast swelling. Illegal if used to "make the weight" in boxing, wrestling, etc.

Wobble board
Balancing board designed to improve ankle, knee and hip coordination.

A-Z of Common Ailments and How to Deal With Them

There are many common or minor injuries or discomforts that can occur in almost any part of the body – if you fall off a bike or wear tight new running shoes, for example. Look here for those common ailments and advice on how to avoid and treat them.

Abrasion
See: Graze.

Athlete's foot
Fungus growing between toes, often picked up in swimming pools and communal showers. Avoid by wearing flip

flops/thonged sandals and drying feet thoroughly. Treat with antifungal powder, liquid or cream and consult doctor if persistent.

Blister

Caused by persistent rubbing against unprotected skin before it can form protective callous. Prevent by slowly building up, and varying, training and by protecting pressure areas (using gloves, plasters or special protectors). To treat blister: (a) clean with antiseptic; (b) use pin sterilized in flame until red hot, then cooled to prick bubble, releasing fluid; (c) leave skin in place, cover with gauze pad, then adhesive tape. If there is spreading red discolouration of skin around blister (or callous), seek medical advice for possible infection. For activity, use a slippery bandage and grease the outside of tape with soap or "second skin" jelly. Two pairs of socks may prevent recurrence on soles of feet.

Boils

Large bumps on the skin, full of pus. Can be due to dirt or ingrown hair. Do not burst, consult doctor.

Bruise

Blood escaping through damaged area and trapped under skin. Use RICE to restrict swelling. Bruise may travel and appear away from injury (always nearer feet, due to gravity).

Bunion

Bony lump on inside of foot, when big toe points outward toward other toes. Soft sponge pad between it and second toe helps straighten big toe. Arch support with pad under big toe and orthotics may correct flattening of arch due to "rolling over" on inside of foot. If inflamed and painful, use aspirin after activity. Occasionally requires surgery if joint is rigid and won't bend back (hallux rigidus or limitus); may require metatarsal bar on shoes to ease discomfort.

Burn

Caused by heat from flame, or by friction, due to sliding after fall on real or artificial turf, cycle track, etc. Treat as for Graze, below.

Callous

Protective thickening of skin layers where rubbing occurs. Forms over bases of fingers in all games where hand holds instrument (racquet sports, hockey, etc.) but most spectacular in men's gymnastics. Should not be removed – just file off rough edges with pumice stone or emery paper.

Cauliflower ear

Swelling and distortion of ear best treated as soon as it develops by draining of haematoma (blood). Often requires repeat drainage.

Collapse

If showing no obvious signs of injury, check if wearing medic-alert disc (used by diabetics, for example). If occurs after competition, is often due to low blood pressure.

If occurs during activity, this must be taken very seriously. Check rectal temperature. See: Heat/Hot weather, Hypothermia, Dehydration. Under 35 years of age: most commonly hypertrophic cardiomyopathy or valve disease. Over 35: coronary heart disease. See: Post-race collapse.

Corn

Hard pad of skin over pressure area having small fluid sac below to allow hard pad to slide back and forth without damaging tissue underneath. If torn and infected, seek medical advice. Corn pads spread load away from pressure point. Claw toes and bunions should be treated and shoes adjusted to fit comfortably.

Cramp

Involuntary shortening of muscle. Exact cause unknown, but poor coordination, poor blood supply, chilling (e.g., while swimming) or excessive salt loss (from extreme sweating) may have effect. Stretch muscle and massage firmly. Some drugs may help, so consult doctor. Sports people can be seen eating bananas during competition. They do this for energy, though some believe the potassium in bananas may prevent cramp.

Cuts

Stop bleeding by pressing with clean cloth (ironed handkerchief is virtually sterile) or fingers. Elevate injured area if possible. Then use cold, running water to clean out dirt, grit, etc. Dab on antiseptic. If shallow, cover with gauze and adhesive tape; if deep, bring edges together with adhesive stitches (See: Steristrip p. 31) or see doctor.

Faintness

Warning all is not well. Sit with head between knees or lie down. Warm down after long run to avoid feeling faint again once you stand up. If occurs during activity, must be taken seriously – contact doctor. See: Post-race collapse.

Graze

When skin is scraped off after a fall on rough or hard surface. Clean with running water, dry and apply antiseptic ointment if available; leave uncovered if possible (plaster keeps area moist, allowing bacteria to grow).

Groin itch/Jock rot/Jock itch

Infection in the groin caused by fungus. Ensure underclothes are clean and changed regularly; dry area well. Treat as athlete's foot, above. Beware: Some lotions sting when applied!

Hyperthermia

Hyperthermia usually occurs in faster, fitter runners and repetition sprint games like soccer. Collapse before the finish of a marathon is likely to be hyperthermia. Must take rectal temperature, as forehead, mouth or ear temperature might be misleading. Ice cooling and replacement of intravenous fluids essential. See: Post-race collapse.

Muscle imbalance

To move a joint, one muscle shortens as its partner lengthens. If one is stronger, causing an imbalance, strains occur. Sometimes result of enthusiastic but poorly scheduled weight-training. Isokinetic machines can measure this balance at different speeds of movement to check whether training should be low loads with high repetitions or high loads with low repetitions. Consult coach.

Poison Ivy

Nasty, itchy rash after contact with poison ivy plant. Wash, apply calamine lotion. Consult doctor.

Post-race collapse

Usually occurs in long-distance events, such as marathon, because leg muscles stop working and stop pumping blood back up to the heart. Blood pressure falls. Make the victim lie down and raise feet. Check rectal temperature in case of hyperthermia. See: Hyperthermia.

Scrape

See: Graze.

Sprung rib

The lower ribs in the rib cage (numbered 9, 10, 11 and 12 by the medical profession) are called floating ribs and may, on impact, flick over the adjoining rib. Rib number 9 is particularly prone to do this. Very painful and quite debilitating. Rest and/or injection required.

Stitch/Side stitch

Common pain under ribs when running. Stop, take deep breaths; when settled, continue.

Supination

See: Pronation.

Turf burn

See: Graze.

Verruca

Wart on foot. The weight of the body makes wart grow inward. Caused by virus. Spread by contact, especially in showers and swimming pools. Consult doctor. Treat with chemicals or freezing gases; wear rubber swimsocks to prevent spreading to others. Use flip flops/thong sandals in shower.

Winding

To counteract the effect of a low punch or impact on the stomach, take short breaths, followed by long breaths to relax muscles. Discomfort should disappear after a few minutes.

Warts

Viral infection on skin. Difficult to remove. The treatments include stringent chemicals, freezing gases to burn out. May just disappear with time.

3

Top-to-Toe Guide to Injuries

DIAGNOSIS, CAUSE, TREATMENT AND TRAINING

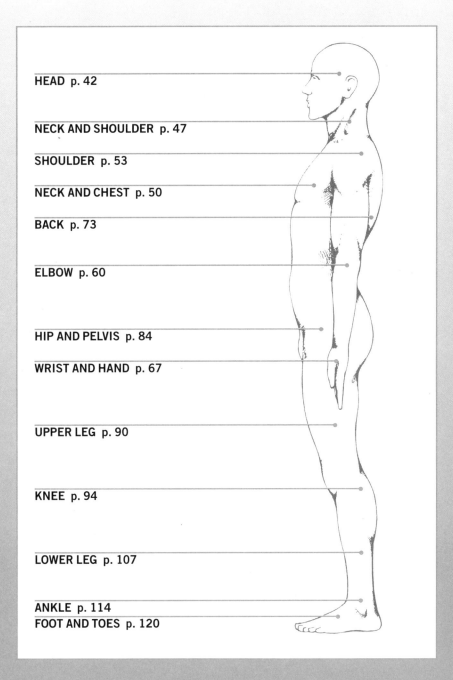

HOW TO USE THIS SECTION

Talk to doctors, and they will insist that there are no such things as sports injuries – just injuries in general. After all, a doctor will treat an ankle sprained from a fall on the stairs in the same way as an ankle injured while playing basketball. What we do here is relate most injuries to sports as these are so common. What we also do is tell you how to recover from your injury – and that will help a painter/decorator who has tennis elbow, as much as a tennis player who has the same injury.

Every effort has been made to cover all the most common sports injuries in this section. Fractures and traumatology, however, have not been covered as they require immediate medical attention. If you cannot identify your injury, or if it does not respond to the treatment indicated, you must seek medical aid.

This section is the central part of the guide and tells you:

- **How to identify your injury**
- **What has produced it**
- **What you can do to help yourself and**
- **What are the likely medical treatments.**

1 Look up the part of the body that you have injured under the headings: Head, Neck and Shoulder, Neck and Chest, Shoulder, Elbow, Wrist and Hand, Back, Hip and Pelvis, Upper Leg, Knee, Lower Leg, Ankle, Foot and Toes. If you do not find the area of injury in the first part you try, look in one adjacent.

2 Now find the painful area or areas marked on the diagram that most nearly matches your pain. Pain indicated on a diagram on the right side of the body also, of course, refers to similar pain on the left side.

3 THIS IS THE CRUCIAL POINT OF THE SELF-DIAGNOSIS. You may find two or three possibilities, so a special test, often with a diagram, will help to identify your specific injury. You may have to try out all the possibilities to ensure correct diagnosis.

Diagnosis/Symptoms

An area around a joint may be painful for several reasons: the muscle and tendons may have been injured, or the joint and its ligaments may have been damaged. To test muscles and tendons, you must make the muscle work without letting the joint move. You do this by trying to make a particular movement but, at the same time, blocking that movement with your opposite hand or arm, the wall, furniture or a friend. This is called **resisted movement.**

To test a joint, you must stop the muscles working (which is harder to do) but still get the joint to move. A good example is getting a friend to lift your arm, rather than using the muscles of that arm. Let the arm go limp, and then get a friend to lift it. This is called **passive movement.**

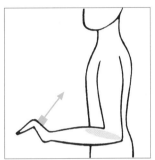

RESISTED MOVEMENT:
To test muscles and tendons

The arrow indicates the direction of the attempted movement. The block under the arrow shows the point at which you must prevent this movement from taking place. The green lines show where the pain will be felt.

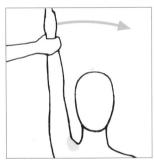

PASSIVE MOVEMENT:
To test joints and ligaments

Take arm as far as you can in the direction indicated by the arrow. The arm may hurt early in the movement or only right at the end. The ligaments may require a little force applied at the end of the movement to show that they are damaged. Never try to show how much pain you can stand. If it hurts, it hurts for a reason. When you see the hand of another person in a diagram, it is a clue that this is a passive movement.

NOTE

- In the few illustrations that have neither a block nor someone else's hands, you should make the movement yourself.
- If these tests do not confirm your injury, try the next possible diagnosis.

Cause

The physical origins of the injury will be given and may indicate that you should alter your technique and training in order to avoid the injury in future.

Treatment

Self: These are ways in which you can help yourself.

Medical: This section is aimed at qualified medical staff and lists some treatments available from doctors.

Training and Rehabilitation

Some doctors will diagnose what is wrong, advise you to rest and even let you return to sports before you have thoroughly recovered. No two injuries, however, are ever exactly the same, so a recommended rest period is always somewhat arbitrary. This is why the author, Dr Malcolm Read, a sports medicine specialist as well as a doctor, has developed **ladder plans** (Chapter 4) that allow the individual to rehabilitate his or her injury at an appropriate pace.

In this section we refer to the appropriate ladder plan for getting back into training. The ladders are designed to gradually load the injured part more and more without redamaging it. As well as the individual ladder plans, the swimming, rowing, cycling and pattering routines referred to in this section are also included in Chapter 4.

It is important to stop your workout if the pain comes back and lasts 20 seconds or more or if you lose your rhythm. Otherwise just work up to the edge of the pain.

How Much Training?

Some injuries do not hurt again until after the ladder rehabilitation session is over. Monitor how heavy your training was. If your injury hurts after training but is back to normal the next morning, merely maintain your training level, but do not increase it. If it still hurts the next morning, but settles down by midday at the latest, then reduce the load a little. If the injury hurts all next day or beyond, then reduce the load considerably. If you suffer no pain after two training sessions, you may then increase the load.

The Back

Millions of working days are lost each year because of "bad" backs. No other part of the body causes more problems. Yet, with a little thought and care, we could all have better posture, stronger muscles to help support our backs and better techniques to prevent back pain, whether we are in the workplace, a sports hall or collecting groceries at the supermarket. There is a special section devoted to the back. See: Problem backs (p. 78).

Joint pain

Sometimes joint pain is caused by arthritis. This can be due to previous damage or wear and tear from age. Arthritis can also be disease-associated, such as rheumatoid and psoriatic arthritis, or even Lyme disease. The only way to find out is to consult a doctor.

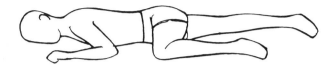

WARNING
Serious injuries on and off the sports field require first-aid treatment. Medical help must be sought at once, so it is always sensible to have the telephone number of the nearest doctor, hospital or medical centre on hand, however casual your level of competition. A mobile telephone, borrowed, if necessary, for the day, is particularly useful for events in a remote or unfamiliar area.

Some basic rules must be followed. In the case of a broken bone (fracture), splint the damaged part to a solid, rigid object and move the victim as little as possible. Cover the victim and keep warm, but do not give anything to drink. If he or she has numbness in the limbs, this could mean a fractured spine. In this case do not move the victim at all. This could only aggravate the injury. Wait for medical assistance. Cover to keep warm and give no liquids or painkillers. See also: Head, Neck and Chest, Shoulder.

If a player loses consciousness because of a blow to the body, place him or her as shown in the diagram above, with clothing loosened. Remove gumshield or false teeth. To keep air passages clear, force chin upward with fingers at angle of jaw.

If a player stops breathing, use artificial respiration techniques such as mouth-to-mouth or mouth-to-nose resuscitation.

NOTE

This is not a first-aid manual. All men and women, as well as their coaches and supporters, should have some knowledge of first aid if they play or attend any sport regularly.

HEAD

This strong, bony box contains the brain and various organs vital to the body's well-being. Injuries may be disfiguring or even disabling, yet too many men and women ignore readily available protections such as eyegoggles, gumshield and helmets. Head guards and helmets must fit properly and be designed for the sport in question. (They must never be used as weapons, like a battering ram.)

Small surface wounds can hide serious problems. A player who cannot remember how he hit his head is suffering from concussion and must not be allowed to continue, however lucid he thinks he is. If the levels of awareness get worse, further medical investigation is imperative.

WARNING

Head and neck injuries can be very serious: (a) if there is numbness or "pins and needles" sensation in arms and legs; or (b) if neither the hand nor foot can be moved. Never move the injured player, even if it means abandoning the game! Get immediate medical help.

A leak of clear fluid from nose or ears suggests a fractured skull. Even a leak of blood from nose or ears should be treated as a fractured skull, but wipe blood away gently to check whether a cut is the cause of bleeding.

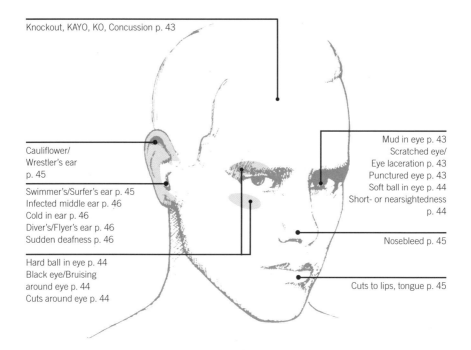

Knockout, KAYO, KO, Concussion p. 43

Cauliflower/
Wrestler's ear
p. 45

Swimmer's/Surfer's ear p. 45
Infected middle ear p. 46
Cold in ear p. 46
Diver's/Flyer's ear p. 46
Sudden deafness p. 46

Hard ball in eye p. 44
Black eye/Bruising
around eye p. 44
Cuts around eye p. 44

Mud in eye p. 43
Scratched eye/
Eye laceration p. 43
Punctured eye p. 43
Soft ball in eye p. 44
Short- or nearsightedness
p. 44

Nosebleed p. 45

Cuts to lips, tongue p. 45

KNOCKOUT, KAYO, KO, CONCUSSION

DIAGNOSIS:
Victim has glazed eyes, is confused, cannot remember events up to and including accident.

CAUSE:
Blow to head

TREATMENT:
Self: Follow first-aid advice. Before moving, remove any gumshield or false teeth. Clear out mouth and nose to allow unobstructed breathing. Then remove from playing area to recover.
Medical: Check airway, give oxygen, neurological signs, consult Glasgow coma scale; x-ray and brain scan.

TRAINING:
No training for 1 week minimum, depending on sport.

NOTE

Concussion has occurred if the person:
- has been unconscious, even for a few seconds;
- does not know what was going on;
- does not speak, get up or open eyes at once;
- was reeling, unable to stand still;
- went into spasms;
- was giddy, threw up or had double vision.

Test for concussion by asking day, month, year; name of opponent in match; the score; walking a line "heel and toe".

Even if players insist they are OK, judgment is often affected. The coach/trainer might have to overrule player, insisting that he or she leaves field/stadium.

Eyes

WARNING

If you wear glasses for sports, they must be unbreakable. Contact lenses will give good all-round vision. Many types of protective goggles (including ones that can be worn over glasses) are now available. Consult eye specialist.

MUD IN EYE

TREATMENT:
Self: Wash eye out with water or, better, salt-water solution (1 teaspoon salt to 1 pint or half litre water), or eye drops.
Medical: Eyebath.

TRAINING:
Continue as usual. Use protective goggles where appropriate.

SCRATCHED EYE/EYE LACERATION

TREATMENT:
Self: Wash eye out with salt-water solution (See: Mud in Eye). Cover with gauze pad. See doctor.
Medical: Antibiotic cream or drops.

PUNCTURED EYE

TREATMENT:
Self: See doctor at once.
Medical: Remove foreign body. Monitor for problems appearing in other eye, refer for ophthalmic opinion.

TRAINING:
Continue as usual, using protective goggles or masks.

WARNING
Check equipment regularly, especially fencing masks, etc.

SOFT BALL IN EYE

Particularly dangerous with small balls in squash, etc., which fit eye socket.

TREATMENT:
Self: Check for clouded vision, bruising. Seek medical advice.
Medical: Check eye lens and for blood in anterior chamber. Check possible blow-out fracture of eye-socket bones.

TRAINING:
Continue as usual. Wear protective goggles.
See: Squash (Chapter 5).

HARD BALL IN EYE

TREATMENT:
Self: Check that all eye movements – up, down, side to side – are normal, with no double or clouded vision. Check bones around eye for fracture. Apply ice pack. Seek medical advice.
Medical: Check for clouded vision, fractures. Broken bone below eye can trap eye muscle, causing double vision later. Check eye lens and for blood in anterior chamber.

TRAINING:
Continue as usual, wearing appropriate head and eye guards.

BLACK EYE/BRUISING AROUND EYE

TREATMENT:
Self: Press ice pack to affected area. Bruising may spread down beneath eye and even cross to other side over next 24-48 hours. Use enzyme cream after 48 hours.

TRAINING:
Continue as usual.

CUTS AROUND EYE

TREATMENT:
Self: Press on edges of wound to stop bleeding. Draw edges together with plaster or butterfly bandage.
Medical: Remove from field of play. As above. Use 1:10,000 adrenalin swab or Embucrylate, cover before return to action. Surgical sutures.
See: Boxing (Chapter 5).

SHORT- OR NEARSIGHTEDNESS

See: Boxing (Chapter 5).

Nose

See: Flu, Hay fever, Head colds
(Chapter 1).

NOSEBLEED

CAUSE:
Usually direct blow, sometimes infection.

TREATMENT:
Self: Keeping head upright, pinch
nostrils together, immediately below bony
part, for 5-10 minutes until blood clots.
If bleeding continues, see doctor.
Medical: Possibly adrenaline. Ice pack.
Check for nose fracture. Check to see if
nasal passages are open. Surgery if
required. If cause is infection, use
antibiotics.

MOUTH AND TEETH

WARNING

Never play sports with false teeth in
place; if dislodged they could cause
choking. Never chew gum for same
reason. Always wear gumshield in sports
where facial blows are possible. Facial
grids attached to helmet also reduce
injury.

CUTS TO LIPS, TONGUE

TREATMENT:
Self: Use ice and compress if possible.
Medical: Stitches may be necessary, but
cuts usually heal easily without.

Ears

CAULIFLOWER/ WRESTLER'S EAR

DIAGNOSIS:
Swollen, painful ear.

CAUSE:
Blood seeps into cartilage, which swells
up, due to blow or rubbing, as in martial
arts, boxing or rugby scrum.

TREATMENT:
Self: Ice pack; compress firmly with
bandage around head. After 48 hours
use enzyme cream.
Medical: Early on, use drainage. NSAIDs.
Later, plastic surgery.

TRAINING:
Continue as usual. Can be prevented in
some sports by wearing protective
headgear or bandaging with tape around
head and ears.

SWIMMER'S/SURFER'S EAR

DIAGNOSIS:
Earache or soreness in outer ear canal
suffered by swimmers, surfers. Hurts to
move ear.

CAUSE:
Persistent wetness. Reaction to salt,
chlorine. Repeated rubbing or scratching
of ear. Over-enthusiastic use of cotton
wool buds.

TREATMENT:
Self: Dry ears thoroughly. Prevent by
using ear plugs, drop of olive oil in ears
before long session in water.
Medical: Antibiotic/cortisone eardrops.

INFECTED MIDDLE EAR

DIAGNOSIS:
Pain deep in ear. moving outer ear does not hurt. Temperature may be raised. Sticky, smelly discharge may appear.

CAUSE:
Infection of eardrum and middle ear. May be due to tooth, mouth or throat infection.

TREATMENT:
Self: Painkillers.
Medical: Antibiotics.

TRAINING:
If temperature and resting pulse normal, continue exercise on land. If discharge from ear, do not swim until given permission by doctor. If grommets have been put in, check with doctor. Probably OK to swim.

COLD IN EAR

DIAGNOSIS:
Fuzzy hearing, maybe pain, especially when flying or diving. There may be crackles and pops but no temperature.

CAUSE:
Glue-like mucus from cold in middle ear clogs eardrum.

TREATMENT:
Self: Pop ears by holding nose then swallowing hard repeatedly, with mouth closed. Chew gum. Blow up balloons. Breathe in menthol inhalation.
Medical: Nasal and ear decongestants. Serious competitors should avoid using decongestants containing drugs on banned lists.

TRAINING:
Avoid sudden changes in pressure (diving, flying).

DIVER'S/FLYER'S EAR

DIAGNOSIS:
Pain in ear due to change of air pressure when diving, scuba diving, flying, etc. Treat as for Cold in ear, above.

SUDDEN DEAFNESS

DIAGNOSIS:
Really does occur all of a sudden, sometimes accompanied by dizziness.

CAUSE:
Ruptured drum in middle ear from loud noise, sudden severe increase in pressure (as in high diving, scuba diving); occasionally disease of arteries in elderly. Occurs cumulatively in sports such as shooting if proper earmuffs or earplugs not used. Also from playing or listening to loud music.

TREATMENT:
Self: See doctor within 48 hours.
Medical: Surgical repair of drum or round window.

TRAINING:
Continue as usual, but ensure proper ear protection if shooting; clear catarrh before diving using menthol crystals. Do not use potent nosedrops for more than 4 days. No swimming until cleared by doctor.

NECK AND SHOULDER

Although this is the weakest link in the body, few athletes carry out the proper exercises to strengthen the muscles that support the neck and shoulders. All the vital connections between the head and body pass through this area, and a fractured neck can mean permanent paralysis.

Thankfully, foul play such as dropping the scrum in Rugby Union has been recognized as highly dangerous, so the incidence of fractures has fallen. Paralysis is caused by forced flexion of the neck. One of the most common causes of permanent paralysis is from diving into water that is too shallow. Always check depth before diving. If in doubt, just slide into the water.

WARNING

Neck pains after a heavy fall, car crash, etc., must be checked by doctor. (See also Serious Injuries and Head warnings, (pp. 40 and 42).

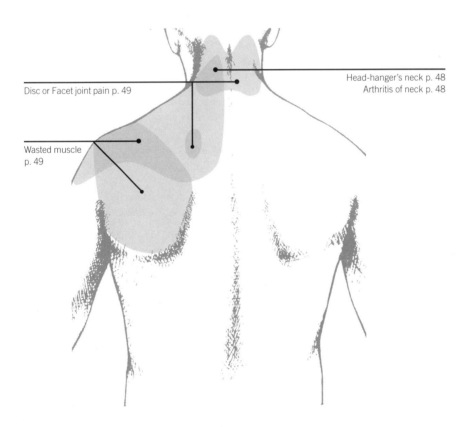

Disc or Facet joint pain p. 49

Head-hanger's neck p. 48
Arthritis of neck p. 48

Wasted muscle
p. 49

HEAD-HANGER'S NECK

DIAGNOSIS:
Although neck can be moved in all directions, it aches, especially when person looks up and down.

CAUSE:
Strain on muscles and ligaments attached to bottom of skull, especially from jobs which involve typing, drawing, etc., all day.

TREATMENT:
Self: Apply warmth. Correct posture. Use painkillers. See: Home and Workplace (p. 156) and Back (p. 73).
Medical: Ultrasound. Shortwave diathermy. Cortisone injection of facet joints or myofascial trigger spot.

TRAINING:
Normal general fitness routine.

ARTHRITIS OF NECK
(Cervical spondylitis/Spondylosis of neck)

DIAGNOSIS:
All neck movements pain free until limit of range is reached on one or both sides. Test as shown in diagrams. (Check also Disc or Facet joint pain – see below).

CAUSE:
Arthritis. May be disease type but usually of the wear-and-tear variety.

TREATMENT:
Self: Painkillers. Exercise neck regularly with slow, gentle nodding, stretching backward and forward and from side to side and turning left and right.
Medical: NSAIDs. Shortwave diathermy. Traction. Manipulation. Inject facet joints.

TRAINING:
Normal general fitness routine, but avoid games that involve violent twisting of neck (rugby, football, wrestling). Sports involving overhead arm action (tennis, badminton) or neck extension (cricket fielder) may present problems.
See: Home and Workplace (p. 156).

DISC OR FACET JOINT PAIN

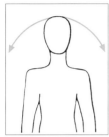

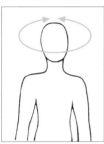

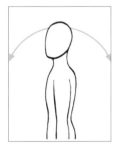

DIAGNOSIS:
Range of neck movements limited and painful (but not all movements painful).
Test as shown in diagrams but not when acutely sore.
Exaggerated nodding and side-to-side movements can also bring on headaches or pain in shoulder, arm, hand, back or chest.

CAUSE:
Whiplash injury. Neck twisted, doing something active or even sleeping. Bones and/or disc in neck move out of proper alignment.

TREATMENT:
Self: Painkillers. Wide, self-supportive collar of folded newspaper wrapped in scarf then tied firmly around neck. At night, tie loop around centre of pillow to make butterfly shape which will support head, or use special pillows.
Medical: Manipulation. Traction. Injection of facet joints. Soft or plastic collar. Painkillers and muscle relaxants. Nerve root block. If pain goes down arm, with evidence of weak muscles, problem can persist for 4-12 weeks whatever treatment used. Patience essential.

TRAINING:
Avoid twisting head; otherwise carry on with normal general fitness routine unless it brings on pain. Bike routine recommended (p. 131).
See: Home and Workplace (p. 156).

WASTED MUSCLE

DIAGNOSIS:
Area looks hollow, flattened.

CAUSE:
Irritation of nerve; muscle does not work, loses tone and strength.

TREATMENT:
Self: Consult doctor.
Medical: Check for disc problems or nerve degeneration. Surgery.

TRAINING:
Occurs in overhead sports such as handball, tennis. Consult doctor before training.

NECK AND CHEST

Since this is where the heart and lungs live, it is potentially the most dangerous area for self-diagnosis. While recent activity might seem to be the reason for a sudden pain here, other problems may well be the cause.

WARNING

Constant pain in the centre or left side of the chest needs urgent attention, especially if also felt in the arms, neck and/or back, particularly if combined with faintness, shortness of breath, cold sweat or fatigue. If there is a stabbing pain when breathing in, check with doctor as this could be result of lung infection, injured ribs or spine.

NOTE

If you have a temperature, stop all training. No sporting injury (apart from dehydration) makes your temperature rise. Resume training only when feeling completely well again.

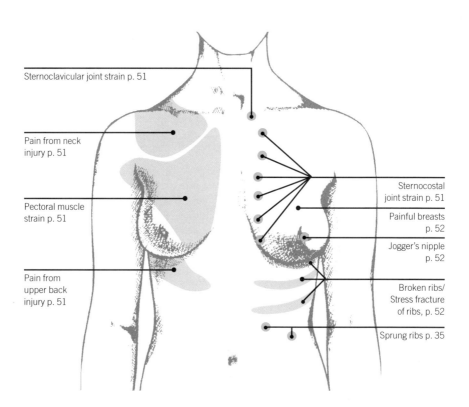

Sternoclavicular joint strain p. 51

Pain from neck injury p. 51

Pectoral muscle strain p. 51

Pain from upper back injury p. 51

Sternocostal joint strain p. 51

Painful breasts p. 52

Jogger's nipple p. 52

Broken ribs/ Stress fracture of ribs, p. 52

Sprung ribs p. 35

PAIN FROM NECK INJURY/BURNER/STINGER

DIAGNOSIS:
Carry out diagnostic tests for Neck and Shoulder injuries. Could run down arm.

TREATMENT:
Self: As for Disc or Facet joint pain.
Medical: Referral pain to 4th cervical root.

PAIN FROM UPPER BACK INJURY

DIAGNOSIS:
Carry out diagnostic tests for Back injuries.

TREATMENT:
Medical: Rib spring negative.

STERNOCLAVICULAR JOINT STRAIN

DIAGNOSIS:
Bony knob at top and side of breastbone tender to pressure; pain may travel up front of neck towards ear. All shoulder movements cause pain in bony knob.

CAUSE:
Strain on joint where collarbone and breastbone meet.

TREATMENT:
Self: Painkillers. Rest arm. If breastbone sticks out further than bony knob, consult doctor immediately.
Medical: NSAIDs. Ultrasound, laser. Cortisone injection. Posterior subluxation may compress major vessels requiring surgery. Check for systemic inflammatory arthropathies.

TRAINING:
Normal general fitness routine; avoid using arm until tenderness goes.

STERNOCOSTAL JOINT STRAIN

DIAGNOSIS:
Tender to pressure over rib joints, about 2 in. (5 cm.) from midline of breastbone; may even feel like lump (as in women's breasts) or cause pain when breathing deeply in and out, slouching, twisting or turning. Pain may occur on one or both sides.

CAUSE:
Strain on hinge joint of rib with breastbone.

TREATMENT:
Self: Painkillers. Rest. Avoid slouching, deep breaths. May take time to heal and can recur.
Medical: NSAIDs. Laser, ultrasound. Cortisone injections. (Tietze syndrome.)

TRAINING:
Normal general fitness routine, but avoid push-ups, weight training using arms.

PECTORAL MUSCLE STRAIN (Pectoral)

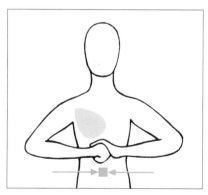

DIAGNOSIS:
Muscles tender to touch, especially at top front of arm. Elbows out, push hands

together across chest; pain confirmed in bust muscles.

CAUSE:
Severe strain, often in martial arts.

TREATMENT:
Self: RICE. Avoid lifting and carrying heavy objects with elbows out (as in lifting a tray). See stretching exercise 3 (p. 10).
Medical: Ultrasound. Interferential. Cross-frictional massage.

TRAINING:
Normal general fitness routine. Isometric exercise against other hand as in diagnostic test. See General muscle ladder (p.132), with push-ups, press-ups. Start with hands at shoulder width; later, move them wider apart as condition improves. Take care with pec deck (pectoralis deck) when weight training.

JOGGER'S NIPPLE
(Men and women)

DIAGNOSIS:
Sore or bleeding nipples.

CAUSE:
Rubbing of clothing on unprotected nipple (male or female); common in distance running, jogging.

TREATMENT:
Self: Leave to heal naturally; allow air to get to affected part if possible, otherwise cover with plaster. Prevent by using petroleum jelly, or tape over with shiny adhesive (smooth plastic adhesive strip) before running; wear clean top.

PAINFUL BREASTS

DIAGNOSIS:
Painful.

CAUSE:
Bouncing, unsupported breasts may be painful after exercise due to torn tissue or friction (See: Jogger's nipple). Blows to breast do not cause cancer; damaged breast fat, however, is very tender, may feel like lump and takes time to heal. Wear supportive sports bra. Check with doctor.

BROKEN RIBS/STRESS FRACTURE

DIAGNOSIS:
Tender after squeezing injured area with hands, compressing and releasing ribs rapidly.

CAUSE:
Crushing or heavy blow, cough, stress fracture.

TREATMENT:
Self: Painkillers. Avoid movements that produce pain. Strapping may be more trouble than it's worth. Takes about 4-6 weeks to heal. Seek medical attention for increased shortness of breath or coughing up blood.
Medical: As above. X-ray. Rowing, canoeing, golf may produce stress fracture. Bone scan participants in these sports.

TRAINING:
Continue as usual if pain tolerable. Check technique with coach if stress fracture.

SHOULDER

This joint has a wide range of movements where the essential strength depends on the condition of muscles and ligaments. Shoulder joint movements also require movement between the shoulder blade and ribs – scapular thoracic, and at the two ends of the collarbone – acromioclavicular (or A/C) and sternoclavicular (or S/C). People often take up activities such as throwing, playing badminton or house-painting without any thought of the problems of acute overuse. Vital nerves and blood vessels are in the armpit, close by the area.

NOTE

The neck can also give shoulder pain, so always check the neck first. See: Neck and Shoulder (p. 47).

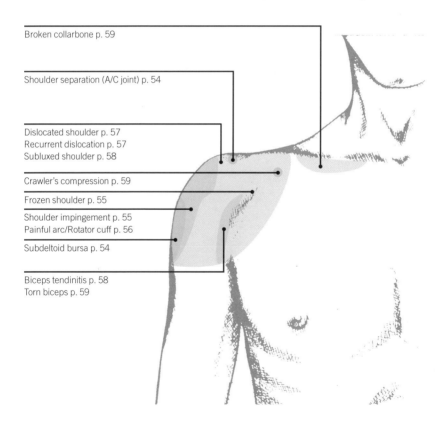

Broken collarbone p. 59

Shoulder separation (A/C joint) p. 54

Dislocated shoulder p. 57
Recurrent dislocation p. 57
Subluxed shoulder p. 58

Crawler's compression p. 59

Frozen shoulder p. 55

Shoulder impingement p. 55
Painful arc/Rotator cuff p. 56

Subdeltoid bursa p. 54

Biceps tendinitis p. 58
Torn biceps p. 59

SHOULDER SEPARATION
(Acromioclavicular joint – A/C joint)

DIAGNOSIS:

Hurts when top of shoulder pressed; may have visible step in shoulder. Hurts to throw a ball. Complete separation may produce fewer problems later on than slight separation.

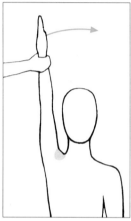

Move raised arm in towards head; pain confirmed near top of shoulder.

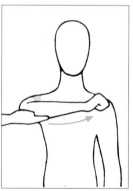

Elbow out, move arm up across chest; pain confirmed near top of shoulder.

CAUSE:

Sprain or rupture of joint ligaments between collarbone and top of shoulder. Usually from fall onto point of shoulder or a lot of overhead work or even sleeping in awkward position with the shoulder and arm drawn across, under chest.

TREATMENT:

Self: Rest. If pain severe, put arm in sling. Avoid carrying heavy weights. Move only within pain-free range.
Medical: NSAIDs. Laser, ultrasound. Cortisone injection. Weight-bearing x-ray. Surgery.

TRAINING:

Normal fitness routine, but avoid throwing overarm, all overhead work, push-ups and carrying heavy weights. See: Badminton, Basketball, Cricket, Cycling, Equestrian sports, Football (American), Netball, Rugby, Squash, Tennis, Volleyball, etc. (Chapter 5).

SUBDELTOID BURSA

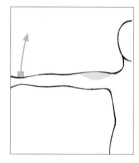

DIAGNOSIS:
Arm must be tested (i.e. arm movement locked) between 45° and horizontal to confirm pain.

CAUSE:
Overuse.

TREATMENT:
Self: RICE. NSAIDs.
Medical: Ultrasound, laser. Cortisone injection.

TRAINING:
Avoid training that flares injury – e.g., press-ups.
See: Tennis (Chapter 5).

SHOULDER IMPINGEMENT
(Subacromial bursa)

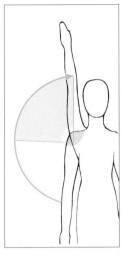

DIAGNOSIS:
Pain occurs when extended arm is brought up from side to a vertical position (especially last 20°). Hurts to throw overarm. Often accompanies other shoulder problems. If diagnosis does not reveal pain but bowling overarm hurts, probably subacromial bursa problem or subluxing shoulder.

CAUSE:
Trapping of bursa or grease bag between armbone and shoulder tip.

TREATMENT:
Self: Rest. NSAIDs.
Medical: NSAIDs.
Cortisone injection. Correct scapulohumeral disassociation and strengthen rotator cuff. Surgery. Shortwave diathermy, interferential.

TRAINING:
Normal general fitness routine, but avoid overhead work. Do not throw overarm; instead throw side or underarm.
See: Badminton, Baseball, Basketball, Cricket, Handball, Netball, Squash, Swimming, Tennis, Volleyball (Chapter 5), Home and Workplace (p. 156).

FROZEN SHOULDER
(Capsulitis)

DIAGNOSIS:
Pain and restricted movement in shoulder joint.

CAUSE:
Wrenched shoulder. Overuse in 50+ age group. May follow injury to disc in neck. Often accompanied by painful arc problems (see below) in young.

TREATMENT:
Self: Immediate support in sling for 48 hours. RICE. NSAIDs. Later, remobilize shoulder gently. Maintain finger and wrist movements at all times.
Medical: Shortwave diathermy. Interferential, mobilization. Cortisone injection. NSAIDs. Surgical manipulation.

TRAINING:
Normal general fitness routine, but swimming and running may be painful; patience needed as joint will flare again if cure not completed. Eventually, carefully graded shoulder strengthening needed.

NOTE
Full recovery from frozen shoulder can take two years, though this may be shortened by medical treatment, usually in three phases:
1 Increasing pain, decreasing movement;
2 Decreased movement, no pain until force movement too far. Frozen shoulder is said to be frozen.
3 Increasing movement. Diabetics take even longer to recover.

PAINFUL ARC/ROTATOR CUFF

DIAGNOSIS:

Pain may occur in any of the following movements: when extended arm is lifted sideways to vertical; when this movement is blocked; and when the arm, out in front (as in diagram), has movement left or right blocked. Pain occurs in arc between 80° and 110°. If little strength can be put against blocked movement, there could be a tear in rotator cuff.

CAUSE:

Overuse of any of four shoulder muscles or poor blood supply in 50+ age group. Poor technique when playing overhead shots. Painting ceilings, polishing tables also triggers pain. Often accompanies shoulder impingement.

TREATMENT:

Self: Rest. Avoid lifting and carrying heavy objects. Avoid work above shoulders. Note: Diabetics usually take much longer to heal.

Medical: Deep friction massage. Laser, ultrasound. Cortisone injection. Work on rotator cuff strength and scapulohumeral disassociation. MRI if torn muscle suspected. Complications such as calcium in tendon or a rupture may need surgery.

TRAINING:

Normal general fitness routine. Keep arms in shape by using spring or elastic band resistance. Follow General muscle ladder (p. 132). Use block test to the edge of pain, follow Rule of 7 (p.131).

See: Home and Workplace (p. 156), Badminton, Basketball, Handball, Netball, Squash, Swimming, Volleyball (Chapter 5).

DISLOCATED SHOULDER

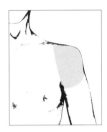

DIAGNOSIS:
Shoulder looks square; arm cannot be lifted outward from side. (See: Recurrent Dislocation of Shoulder.)

CAUSE:
Severe wrench or fall causes armbone (humerus) to dislocate from shoulder socket.

TREATMENT:
Self: Do not attempt to do anything yourself – except put in sling. Seek medical advice as fractures may complicate injury.
Medical: X-ray to exclude possibility of fracture to arm or socket. Reset: may need anaesthetic. Usually anterior dislocation, posterior easy to miss. Sling.

TRAINING:
Keep shoulder immobilized about one month. Heels (p. 144, step 5). Bicycle, running, step, rowing machine. Later, swimming, going gently in the freestyle, butterfly. Seek medical advice. When fully mobile again, begin strengthening of shoulder muscles. Young people will be prone to redislocation; those over 40 more to frozen shoulder.

RECURRENT DISLOCATION OF SHOULDER

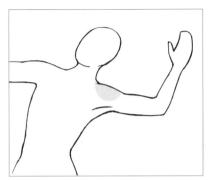

Danger position

In some people, the shoulder dislocates easily and often, especially in the danger position. However, it can also be relocated quite easily.

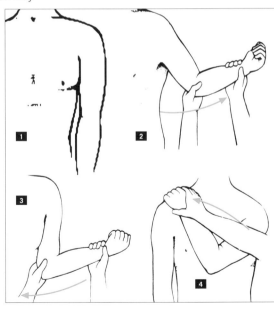

TREATMENT:

Self: Lie face down on couch/table. Let injured arm hang down holding heavy weight. Take time to relax. Standing up, manipulate into place using what is known as Kocher manoeuvre (see diagram). If this doesn't work first time, don't persist; consult doctor.

Medical: Put in place. Check Bankart or Hill-Sachs lesion on x-ray or MRI. Surgery can prevent further dislocation by tightening muscles and ligaments. If it is the preferred arm in throwing or for a racquet sport, early surgery needed.

TRAINING:

Normal general fitness routine once shoulder back in place. Avoid falling on shoulder or above-shoulder racquet work until soreness gone. Gradually build up shoulder muscle strength.

SUBLUXED SHOULDER

CAUSE:

Partial dislocation or unstable shoulder that has been dislocated before. Loose shoulder with lax ligaments.

DIAGNOSIS:

Shoulder jumps in socket. Dead arm after throwing. Pain at times.

TREATMENT:

Self: Avoid throwing, overarm action; strengthen arc muscles. Avoid danger position.

See: Recurrent dislocation.

Medical: If apprehension tests are positive, use isometric and isokinetic strength rehabilitation. Surgery.

TRAINING:

Under professional supervision.

BICEPS TENDINITIS

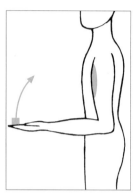

DIAGNOSIS: Palm up, try to lift forearm. Pain confirmed in front of shoulder, although this sign is often absent.

CAUSE:

Overuse of muscle due to carrying, lifting or pulling with elbow bent.

TREATMENT:

Self: RICE. NSAIDs. After 48 hours use frictional massage on tender spot.

Medical: Deep friction massage. Laser, ultrasound. Cortisone injection.

TRAINING:

Normal general fitness routine. Follow General muscle ladder (p. 132). Avoid pulling or carrying with bent elbow or using screwdriver. Build gradually into chin-ups, with hands under bar and biceps curls.

See: Canoeing/Kayaking (Chapter 5).

TORN BICEPS (Popeye arm)

DIAGNOSIS:

As for Biceps tendinitis but accompanied by bruising. Even when relaxed, muscle looks bunched (like Popeye's).

CAUSE:

In older people, lifting too heavy a weight with elbow bent. In younger people, sudden check when lifting heavy weight or making full-blooded move with bent elbow (in wrestling, weightlifting, etc.).

TREATMENT:

Self: RICE. After 1 week start easy stretching to straighten elbow.
Medical: Laser, ultrasound, stretching. As torn ends of tendon usually re-attach further down, surgery rarely required

TRAINING:

Normal general fitness routine. Follow General muscle ladder (p. 132). Build up to chin-ups with hands under bar and biceps curls.

BROKEN COLLARBONE

DIAGNOSIS:

Victim feels bones rubbing together even if break not obviously visible.

CAUSE:

Blow on collarbone or fall.

TREATMENT:

Self: Place arm on injured side in sling. See doctor.
Medical: Sling. Occasionally surgery.

TRAINING:

Normal general fitness routine. Use bicycle one-handed (stationary bike recommended). Pattering (p. 129), then running; make sure calf, thigh and stomach muscles are kept in shape. Shoulder and hand mobility must be maintained at all times. Try supporting elbow on injured side with opposite hand, then waving forearm gently from side to side. estimated 6-8 weeks for bones to knit. When can do 6 push-ups, can ride horse. When can do 10 push-ups, can ride motorbike.

CRAWLER'S COMPRESSION

See: Swimming (Chapter 5).
Medical: This area may also have pain from short head of biceps.

ELBOW

Apart from falls, lack of coordination and overuse produce the majority of injuries in the elbow. This joint, with its associated muscles, also controls wrist and finger movements. As many sports have their own traditional names for particular injuries, the same injury can have several nicknames. What is commonly known as tennis elbow can be caused by an enthusiast at home spending a weekend putting up shelves – using a screwdriver! Pitcher's elbow, from the world of baseball, actually covers several different injuries, all of them caused by different pitching techniques. More often than not, the injury can be cured by correcting the technical fault, in cooperation with a good coach.

WARNING

• Children who injure this joint may disturb growing points, causing distorted or slow growth. Medical treatment is essential.

• Persistent pins and needles in the hand below a recently injured elbow or lack of pulse at the wrist are danger signals. Seek medical treatment at once.

FRONT

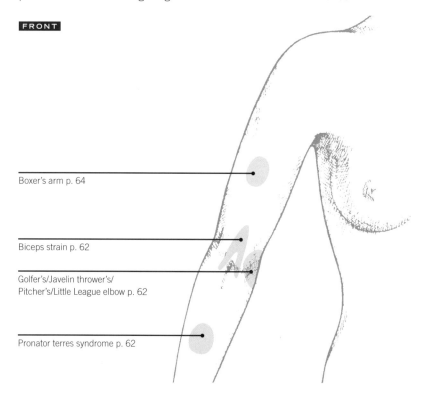

Boxer's arm p. 64

Biceps strain p. 62

Golfer's/Javelin thrower's/
Pitcher's/Little League elbow p. 62

Pronator teres syndrome p. 62

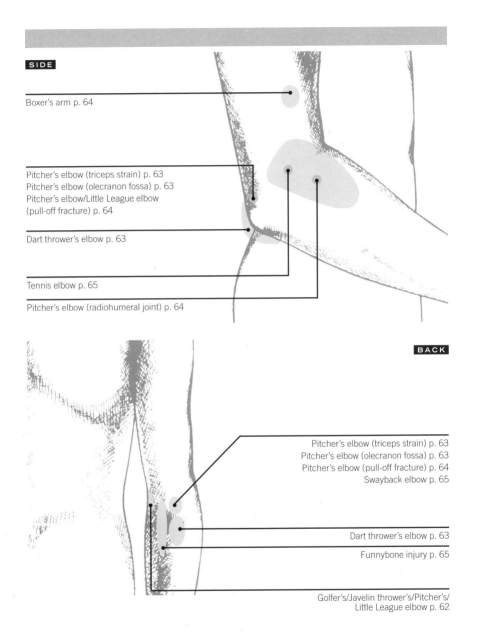

SIDE

Boxer's arm p. 64

Pitcher's elbow (triceps strain) p. 63
Pitcher's elbow (olecranon fossa) p. 63
Pitcher's elbow/Little League elbow
(pull-off fracture) p. 64

Dart thrower's elbow p. 63

Tennis elbow p. 65

Pitcher's elbow (radiohumeral joint) p. 64

BACK

Pitcher's elbow (triceps strain) p. 63
Pitcher's elbow (olecranon fossa) p. 63
Pitcher's elbow (pull-off fracture) p. 64
Swayback elbow p. 65

Dart thrower's elbow p. 63

Funnybone injury p. 65

Golfer's/Javelin thrower's/Pitcher's/
Little League elbow p. 62

BICEPS STRAIN

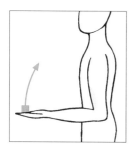

DIAGNOSIS:
With palm up, try to bend elbow. Pain confirmed in elbow or upper arm.

CAUSE:
Strain on biceps muscle (bulging one on front of arm, above elbow) or tendon at elbow.

TREATMENT:
Self: RICE if pain in muscle but NOT if in elbow. Slow to heal on its own. Avoid lifting heavy loads.
Medical: Ultrasound, laser. Frictional massage. Biceps strain very slow to heal in spite of all treatment. Beware adjacent structures.

TRAINING:
Normal general fitness routine, including upper body strength; no forearm bends or press-ups. See: Archery (Chapter 5).

PRONATOR TERRES SYNDROME

DIAGNOSIS:
Gripping friend's hand, try to turn palm down. Resist pressure on tip of middle finger. Pain confirmed in forearm.

CAUSE:
Rare. Technical fault in racquet sports.

TREATMENT:
Self: RICE. Pain may persist for several months. Stretch forearm muscle by forcing tips of fingers back until pain felt

in forearm. Hold, release and repeat.
Medical: Cortisone injection. Surgery.

TRAINING:
Continue as usual unless painful. See: Squash, Tennis (Chapter 5).

GOLFER'S/JAVELIN THROWER'S/ PITCHER'S/LITTLE LEAGUE ELBOW

All occur on or around the bony knob on inner side of elbow. Although injury appears to be produced by different actions, it is the forceful curl of wrist, the pressure from fingertips or the force of the palm down while bending the fingers that puts undue stress on elbow.

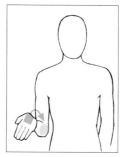

DIAGNOSIS:
Blocking the attempt to twist the palm (so that it faces down) always hurts. With palm up, resist wrist curl, or curl of fingers.
Pain usually, but not always, confirmed round bony knob on inner side of elbow.

CAUSE:
Strain of forearm muscle's tendon at elbow. These muscles curl the wrist and close fingers into fist. Powerful pulling and gripping may strain them and even pull off a piece of bone or damage the growing point in youngsters.

TREATMENT:
Self: RICE, but use ice for only 5 minutes as near nerves. Avoid gripping with the palm facing up, especially using the tips of the fingers for jobs such as pulling up

weeds, polishing small area of shoes, furniture. Stretch fingers backward to start of pain, hold and release. Block as in diagnosis tests. Use Rule of 7 (p. 131). *Medical:* Cross-frictional massage. Laser, ultrasound. NSAIDs. Cortisone injections. Surgery.

TRAINING:
Normal general fitness routine, including upper body strength; no grip strengthening, no wrist curls. See: Golf, Baseball, Track and Field athletics, Tennis (Chapter 5).

PITCHER'S ELBOW (Triceps strain)

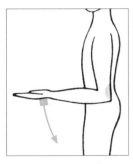

DIAGNOSIS: Palm up, resist attempt to push forearm down to side.

CAUSE:
Too much load on elbow. Can be in "clean" segment of clean and jerk lift in weight lifting; forceful straightening of the elbow, as in throwing, or serving in tennis. Triceps dips, elbow bone may be damaged as well.

TREATMENT:
Self: RICE. Recovers quite quickly.
Medical: Beware avulsion and stress fracture injuries. Ultrasound, laser. Cross-frictional massage. Interferential. NSAIDs. Cortisone injection.

TRAINING:
Normal general fitness routine; no heavy weights until pain free. Avoid triceps curls, dips. See: Baseball, Tennis (Chapter 5).

PITCHER'S ELBOW (Olecranon fossa)

DIAGNOSIS:
Straighten elbow; pain felt when it locks. No pain when bent.

CAUSE:
Repeatedly snapping elbow straight, as in pitching, throwing or karate.

TREATMENT:
Self: RICE.
Medical: Olecranon fossa impingement. Ultrasound. Cortisone injection.

TRAINING:
Normal fitness routine. Maintain movement but avoid 100 per cent snap of throw. When pain is no longer felt on straightening elbow, ease back to full throwing. Take your time, as problem may flare up again. See: Baseball, Squash (Chapter 5).

DART THROWER'S ELBOW (Olecranon bursa)

DIAGNOSIS:
Tender swelling around tip of elbow.

CAUSE:
Repeated flexing of elbow, not necessarily with heavy weight, e.g. in rifle shooting or darts; gout or infection, such as grazed elbow; fall or even beer drinker leaning on bar.

TREATMENT:
Self: RICE. Avoid pressure on elbow. If

elbow looks red, infected, see doctor. *Medical:* Antibiotics if infected; NSAIDs (also for gout); drain fluid; check for uric acid crystals or culture. Cortisone injection.

TRAINING:
Normal training routine. Avoid any exercises that cause more pain in elbow. See: Darts (Chapter 5).

PITCHER'S ELBOW/LITTLE LEAGUE ELBOW (Pull-off fracture)

DIAGNOSIS:
See: Golfer's elbow, above.

CAUSE:
This is same injury as golfer's elbow, but occurs in children where growing point of elbow is at risk. Muscle tears away from bone taking small fragment with it.

TREATMENT:
Self: Rest. Allow some 8 weeks for fragment to re-attach.
Medical: Splinting. Possible surgery.

TRAINING:
Normal fitness routine; consult medical adviser.
See: Baseball (Chapter 5).

PITCHER'S ELBOW (Radiohumeral joint)

DIAGNOSIS:
As for tennis elbow, but more so. Pain also from passive straightening of elbow or full bending of elbow and full twisting of forearm (from palm up to palm down and vice versa). May hurt even at rest.

CAUSE:
Joint strained by snapping elbow straight

as wrist turns palm down, as in baseball pitching, badminton shot at net.

TREATMENT:
Self: RICE. Needs more time to heal than tennis elbow.
Medical: Shortwave diathermy. Interferential. NSAIDs. Cortisone injection. All concurrent with tennis elbow treatment.

TRAINING:
Normal fitness routine. If uncomplicated by tennis elbow, all moves that do not produce pain. Make sure technique is correct. Consult coach.
See: Badminton, Baseball, Tennis (Chapter 5).

BOXER'S ARM

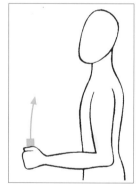

DIAGNOSIS:
Fist clenched, thumb on top, try to lift forearm. Pain confirmed in upper arm.

CAUSE:
Rare. Small spur of bone that develops in some boxers just above elbow is broken off by direct blow.

TREATMENT:
Self: Rest. With extended rest (4-6 weeks), spur will re-attach itself.
Medical: Attachment of ligament of Struther is fractured. Cortisone

injections. Surgical removal.

TRAINING:

Normal fitness routine, including upper body strength; no punching until pain free.

FUNNYBONE INJURY
(Ulnar neuritis)

DIAGNOSIS:

Straightening (flattening) the elbow completely and touching spot on the inside of the elbow knob produces tingling, pain, pins and needles down the forearm, classically into 4th and 5th fingers. Pain may even extend upwards into shoulder, causing wakefulness at night.

CAUSE:

Pressure/damage to nerve, either by blow, regularly leaning on it or overuse of nearby muscles. Pressure may be on ulnar nerve over wrist or heel of hand (pisiform)
See: Pisiform strain.

TREATMENT:

Self: Rest. Avoid pressure on nerve, especially from table edge, car window.
Medical: EMG. Cortisone injection. Surgery.

TRAINING:

Normal fitness routine. Seek medical advice.

SWAYBACK ELBOW

See: Gymnastics (Chapter 5).

TENNIS ELBOW

The most common injury to this joint. Although labelled a tennis complaint, it can occur in the home or the workplace or in any action where the elbow is constantly bending while the hand is gripping, e.g., painting the ceiling with a roller-type brush, canoeing, kayaking, badminton, baseball pitching, tenpin bowling, even flyfishing.

One cause is simply doing too much in a concentrated spell, such as redecorating during the weekend or even improving at a sport, perhaps when adding curve or spin to your throw or stroke. The better you get, the more you need to increase your body's strength to handle this added stress. If you do not, the result is an injury. Another cause in tennis is poor technique, especially on the backhand, or gripping the racquet too tightly with thumb and index finger. Pain and tenderness to the touch occur on the outer side of the elbow and may extend down the forearm.

DIAGNOSIS:

Turning the hand palm up, cocking the wrist and straightening the fingers all cause pain. See drawings overleaf.

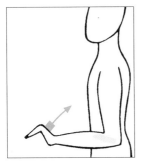

1 Resist cocking wrist backward. Pain confirmed.

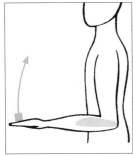

2 Fingers extended, palm down, try to lift forearm with resistance over tips of fingers.

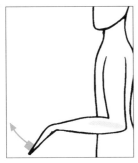

3 Fingers extended downward, resist cocking wrist at fingertips.

CAUSE:

Classic overuse strain where hand drops, wrist twists and arm bends – anything from using screwdriver to playing tennis. Forearm muscles are not strong enough to take strain. Often caused by technical fault or unsuitable equipment.
See Pitcher's elbow (Radiohumeral joint sprain) for complications.

TREATMENT:

Self: RICE. Avoid lifting all objects with palm down. Even writing with thin pen/pencil causes flare-up so use thicker pen/pencils. When doing home improvements, long-handled or powered screwdrivers reduce force required. Try to grip with 3rd, 4th and 5th fingers, relaxing the index finger and thumb. In tennis, do not drop wrist or lead with elbow in backhand. To stretch muscle, face the palms of your hands towards each other. Then turn hands palm down and continue turning bad arm to face palm outward. Curl/bend wrist forward with other hand as far as you can and straighten elbow. Hold 7 seconds, then repeat block tests 1, 2 and 3. Hold to pain for count of 7. Repeat 7 times.
Medical: Laser, ultrasound. Deep friction massage. Cortisone injection. Surgery. If extending the arm feels worse and bending the arm feels better, or if patient wakes at night, then check for radial nerve entrapment.

TRAINING:

Normal fitness routine. When pain free, strengthen forearm with supported wrist curls – with elbow supported, raise and lower wrist while holding 4½ lb (2 kg) weight.
Extra aids: Forearm strapping and tennis elbow supports: act like an outer skeleton and take load off sore spot.
See: Archery, Badminton, Baseball, Canoeing, Golf, Skiing, Squash (Chapter 5), Home and Workplace (p. 156).

WRIST AND HAND

A large area of the brain is reserved to look after this sensitive and vital part, which can handle an activity as delicate as sewing yet act as a weapon in martial arts. As a first-line sensor it comes into contact with objects that may damage and interfere with its fine control. Its many bones may suffer strains and sprains.

WARNING

There are so many bones and joints in fingers and wrists that self-diagnosis of a sprain or break is difficult. Seek medical advice.

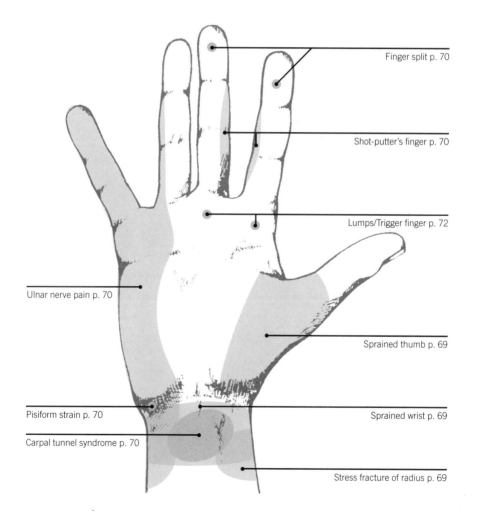

Finger split p. 70

Shot-putter's finger p. 70

Lumps/Trigger finger p. 72

Ulnar nerve pain p. 70

Sprained thumb p. 69

Pisiform strain p. 70

Sprained wrist p. 69

Carpal tunnel syndrome p. 70

Stress fracture of radius p. 69

WRIST AND HAND

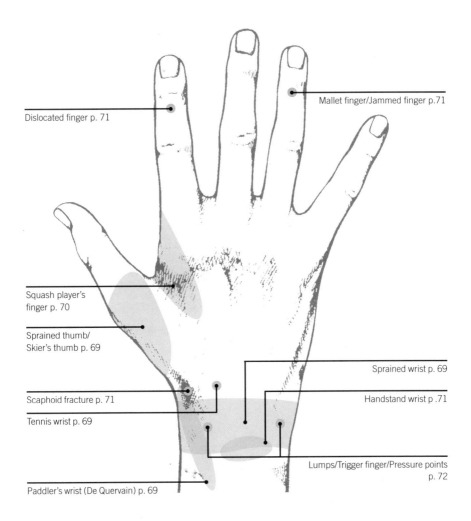

Dislocated finger p. 71

Mallet finger/Jammed finger p.71

Squash player's finger p. 70

Sprained thumb/Skier's thumb p. 69

Scaphoid fracture p. 71

Tennis wrist p. 69

Sprained wrist p. 69

Handstand wrist p .71

Lumps/Trigger finger/Pressure points p. 72

Paddler's wrist (De Quervain) p. 69

SPRAINED WRIST

DIAGNOSIS:

Moving wrist in any direction painful; pain shows up sometimes in small, sometimes in larger, movements.

CAUSE:

Usually twist or fall, spraining linings and ligaments.

TREATMENT:

Self: RICE. Strap using "cock up" splint. If unavailable, use 1-2 in. (5 cm.) stretch elastic bandage, place wrist in "cocked" position, make tight fist, relax it, then strap wrist in that position. When better, use elastic wrist support. NSAIDs. Continue pain free wrist movements.

Medical: As above. Shortwave diathermy.

TRAINING:

Normal general fitness routine. Wrist movement should be supported 2-4 weeks. Work up to, not through, pain.

TENNIS WRIST

DIAGNOSIS:

Pain mainly on bending wrist backward, though other movements may hurt. Tenderness in wrist at back but beneath hand bones of second and third fingers.

CAUSE:

Often through switching to Western grip at tennis. Wrist bones hit together when fully extended at impact.

TREATMENT:

Self: Switch to semi-Western or even standard grip.

Medical: As above. Try cortisone injection.

STRESS FRACTURE OF RADIUS

See: Gymnastics (Chapter 5).

PADDLER'S WRIST (De Quervain)

See: Home and Workplace (p. 156), Canoeing, Rowing (Chapter 5).

SPRAINED THUMB/ SKIER'S THUMB

DIAGNOSIS:

Tip of thumb can be moved but lower joint hurts on all movements, especially pushing outward. May show swelling and bruising.

CAUSE:

Forceful wrenching of lower thumb joint.

WARNING

If bones fracture so that thumb is displaced, surgery (pinning) will be necessary. This may happen when a skier falls – the strap on the poles wrenches thumb. Thermoplastic splint will protect for skiing.

See: Skiing (Chapter 5).

TREATMENT:

Self: RICE (compression essential). Strap from wrist down to sore joint with 1-2 in. (5 cm.) elastic support, also covering palm. High sling helps reduce swelling over 48 hours. Anti-bruise cream. Unstrap after 48 hours and gently try opening fist, then closing with fingers over thumb; re-bandage. Support thumb 4-6 weeks if there is any possibility of it being bent backward in everyday activities – lifting, carrying.

Medical: Check for Bennett fracture.

NSAIDs. Laser, ultrasound. Enzyme creams after 48 hours.

TRAINING:
Normal general fitness routine; support thumb if necessary. Avoid ball-handling games using large ball (football, basketball) and martial arts until better.

SHOT-PUTTER'S FINGER

See: Track and Field Athletics (Chapter 5).

SQUASH PLAYER'S FINGER

See: Squash (Chapter 5).

ULNAR NERVE PAIN

DIAGNOSIS:
Pins and needles or pain down 4th and 5th fingers.

CAUSE:
Nerve pain. Consult doctor.
See: Elbow (p. 60). Pressure at wrist may also damage ulnar nerve as it passes near butt of hand. See: Cycling (Chapter 5).

PISIFORM STRAIN

DIAGNOSIS:
Prominent bony lump on palm of wrist little finger side; sore if pushed sideways. May have ulnar nerve pain as well.

CAUSE:
Pressure on bone from sporting implement.

TREATMENT:
Self: Check technique or implement with coach to correct cause of problem.

Medical: Correct cause of problem with coach. Inject cortisone into pisihamate ligaments.
See: Golf, Tennis, Squash (Chapter 5).

CARPAL TUNNEL SYNDROME

DIAGNOSIS:
Pain in palm, thumb, index and middle fingers; sometimes in wrist, forearm and upper arm. Pain is sufficient to wake you at night. Tapping wrist on the skin creases on palm side may cause shooting sensation in hand (Tinel test). Thumb muscles may weaken.

CAUSE:
Pressure on nerve passing into wrist, from overuse, pregnancy or disease such as under-active thyroid.

TREATMENT:
Self: Keep wrist higher than elbow. Seek medical advice.
Medical: Diuretics. Cortisone injection. Surgery especially if thenar eminence wasting. Correct thyroid problems.

TRAINING:
Continue as usual unless painful. Repeated pressure may flare condition.

FINGER SPLIT

DIAGNOSIS:
Split in skin.

CAUSE:
Overuse. Sometimes a grip on a bat or racquet prevents finger sliding, so pressure causes split in skin.

TREATMENT:
Self: Tape fingers before training or playing.

MALLET FINGER/JAMMED FINGER

DIAGNOSIS:
Inability to straighten last joint of finger.

CAUSE:
Tendon that straightens the tip of finger has been torn off.

TREATMENT:
Self: RICE. Use pencil or short piece of wood as splint under finger. Strap so last joint is straight, or cocked backward if possible. Seek medical advice.
Medical: Splint into extension.

TRAINING:
Continue as usual, with splint in place if possible.

HANDSTAND WRIST

DIAGNOSIS:
Back of wrist aches when hand forced back as in handstand.

CAUSE:
Inadequate wrist extendibility compresses bones in wrist.

TREATMENT:
Self: Do not overwork wrist; gradually build up handstands, press-ups. Try turning hands outward or inward during handstands to find position that causes less pain. Rest.
Medical: Rest. Shortwave diathermy.

TRAINING:
Continue as usual, but build up handstand work gradually.
See: Gymnastics (Chapter 5).

SCAPHOID FRACTURE

DIAGNOSIS:
Pain in hollow between two thumb tendons on back of wrist.

CAUSE:
Fall on hand.

TREATMENT:
Self: Seek medical advice.
Medical: Difficult to diagnose even with x-ray (if in doubt, use a scan). Cast. Splint.

TRAINING:
Continue as usual, if possible with cast.

DISLOCATED FINGER

DIAGNOSIS:
Tip of finger points backward. Lump in front of end joint.

TREATMENT:
Self: Following only applicable to end joint; any others, seek medical help.
1 As soon as possible, pull, as if trying to stretch fingertip out from rest of finger; joint will slide back into place.
2 If unsuccessful, stop, seek medical help.
3 Strap injured finger to next finger for 24 hours.
4 NSAIDs.
5 After 24 hours, gently move finger towards making a fist (warming in hot water, wearing protective rubber glove, may help).
6 Swelling may continue for months.
Medical: As for self-treatment. Wax baths.

TRAINING:

Continue as usual, but strap joint for 3 weeks for ball-handling or martial arts sports.

LUMPS/TRIGGER FINGER

DIAGNOSIS:

Hard or rubbery lumps, usually on back of wrist; can be on any finger or wrist joint. Up to 95 per cent of lumps are what are called synovial cysts. If occurring at base of fingers this may be a thickening of tendon, which leads to finger staying bent, before flicking out suddenly with jerk, which is why it is often called Trigger finger.

CAUSE:

Weak lining of joint bulges with yellow, jelly-like, joint-lubricating fluid.

TREATMENT:

Self: Leave alone.

Medical: Pressure. Drain with needle. Injection cortisone or surgery to trigger finger.

TRAINING:

Continue as usual.

PRESSURE POINTS

DIAGNOSIS:

Area tender to pressure or use, usually on back or outside of wrist.

CAUSE:

Weakness in joint linings.

TREATMENT:

Self: Bandage wrist firmly for training or playing.

BACK

While walking on two legs has permitted us to develop those mechanical marvels—the hands, it has also loaded our backs in the upright position. We rarely concern ourselves, however, with posture and deportment, even though more working days are lost from back trouble than any other cause. Correct posture, together with back and stomach muscle strength, can correct 80 per cent of back-care problems, saving many days of pain. As well as covering the diagnosis and treatment of back problems, this section includes some general tips on living and training with them. Don't forget that back injuries may not always be the same. Manipulation may work once but not the next time.

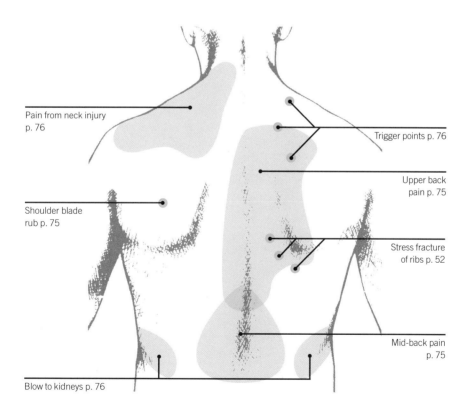

Pain from neck injury p. 76

Trigger points p. 76

Upper back pain p. 75

Shoulder blade rub p. 75

Stress fracture of ribs p. 52

Mid-back pain p. 75

Blow to kidneys p. 76

BACK

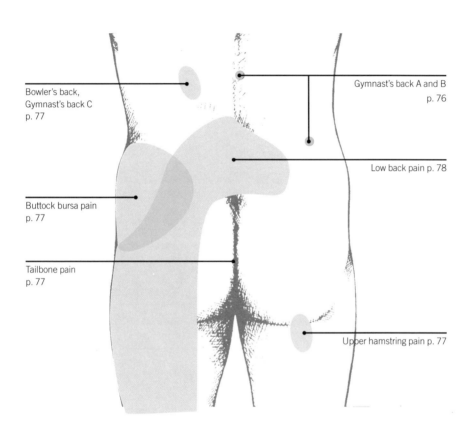

Bowler's back,
Gymnast's back C
p. 77

Gymnast's back A and B
p. 76

Low back pain p. 78

Buttock bursa pain
p. 77

Tailbone pain
p. 77

Upper hamstring pain p. 77

UPPER BACK PAIN (Dorsal)

DIAGNOSIS:
Some or all of the following may produce pain: breathing or coughing; lowering chin onto chest; turning upper body one way rather than another; bending to side. Occasionally pain may be felt in front of chest as well as in back.

CAUSE:
Backbone (facet joint) or its shock absorber in between (the disc) moved out of place, so ligaments are stretched and muscles may cramp.

TREATMENT:
Self: Rest. Seek medical advice. Avoid twisting top half of body and lifting from side. Instead, turn to face object before lifting. Sitting may be easier than lying down, so prop up pillows to form "chairback" on bed. Painkillers. Always use neutral position (see p. 79).
Medical: Rest. Painkillers. Manipulation. Facet joint injections. X-ray. MRI or CT Scan. Note Scheuermann's osteochondritis in adolescents.

TRAINING:
Normal general fitness routine, as long as pain free. Bicycling, ergometric rowing easier and better than running or swimming. No upper body work until better. Otherwise, general training for back (p. 81).
See: Golf, Rowing, Rugby (Chapter 5); Home and Workplace (p. 156).

MID-BACK PAIN

DIAGNOSIS:
Pain may be in loin area, (as for upper back), or when leaning backward.

CAUSE:
(a) Pushing/pulling with rounded back (b) slumping with hollow low back and rounded upper back (c) standing tall but hollowing mid back, which causes an impingement of facet joints.

TREATMENT:
Self: Correct bad posture; use neutral position (p. 79) for life. If caused by over-forcing the back strain position, relax; allow hollow to form in lower spine. Stand with weight towards balls of feet. Rest. Painkillers. Seek medical advice.
Medical: X-ray teenagers as this may be growth problem. Manipulation. Traction.

TRAINING:
Continue as usual if pain free. Maintain back strain position, especially with weights. However, when the muscles you are training tire (so that you start using your back and body to help), it is time to stop. Work on back strength when fit.
See: Home and Workplace (p. 156), Rowing, Rugby (Chapter 5).

SHOULDER BLADE RUB (Subscapular crepitus)

DIAGNOSIS:
Neither shoulder tests (see: Shoulder, p. 53) nor twisting upper body produce pain. But circling shoulder (not arm) is painful and produces grating feeling if flat of hand is placed on shoulder blade.

CAUSE:
Rough underside of shoulder blade rubbing over ribs.

TREATMENT:
Self: Hold shoulders squarely as tense, rounded shoulders will cause pain to flare up.
Medical: Shortwave diathermy. Interferential. Cortisone injection under shoulder blade. Surgery.

TRAINING:
Continue as usual. Ensure square shoulders and non-rounded upper back. See: Golf (Chapter 5).

BLOW TO KIDNEYS

TREATMENT:
Self: Apply ice/cold compress.

TRAINING:
Continue as much as pain allows.

NOTE
If blood appears in urine or pain increases, seek medical advice at once.

PAIN FROM NECK INJURY

Carry out diagnostic tests for Neck and Shoulder injuries (pp. 47, 53).
See: Home and Workplace (p. 156).

TRIGGER POINTS

DIAGNOSIS:
Muscles may be locally tender to touch.

CAUSE:
Often following neck or upper body problems or muscle inflammation.

TREATMENT:
Self: Localized massage

Medical: Stretching. Ultrasound. Acupuncture. Accupressure. Cortisone injection.

Lower back

GYMNAST'S BACK A

DIAGNOSIS:
Pain in midline between bony knobs of spine only when arching backward.

CAUSE:
Bones knocking on each other when back arched in acute angle, known as hyperextension.

TREATMENT:
Self: See: Gymnastics (Chapter 5).
Medical: Laser, ultrasound. Cortisone injection to interspinous ligament. Rarely, surgery.

TRAINING:
See: Gymnastics (Chapter 5).

GYMNAST'S BACK B

DIAGNOSIS:
Pain only in completion of full backward arch. "Swallows" may hurt. Edge of pelvic bone on back tender to pressure, usually one side only.

CAUSE:
Walkovers.

TREATMENT:
Self: See: Gymnastics (Chapter 5).
Medical: Laser, ultrasound. Cortisone injection.

TRAINING:
See: Gymnastics (Chapter 5).

GYMNAST'S BACK C

DIAGNOSIS:
Pain on leaning backward.

CAUSE:
Stress fracture of vertebrae from
extension and twisting movement.

TREATMENT:
Self: For persistent back pain, seek
medical advice.
Medical: Spondylolysis. Scan. SPECT, CT
or MRI. Relative rest. Spondylolisthesis,
x-ray and obliques.
See: Gymnastics (Chapter 5).

TAILBONE PAIN (Coccygitis)

DIAGNOSIS:
Often constant pain, especially sitting
down but sometimes bending forward.
Tip of spine (bones between buttocks)
tender to touch.

CAUSE:
Sitting down suddenly and hard on tip of
spine; may even cause fracture.

TREATMENT:
Self: Sit forward on fleshy part of upper
thighs. Sit on inflatable ring or on gap
between 2 cushions. Painkillers. Healing
often takes more than 4 weeks – be
patient!
Medical: Painkillers. NSAIDs. Cortisone
injection. Very rarely, surgery.

TRAINING:
Normal routine as far as possible, but
avoid rowing and bicycling.
See: Skating (Chapter 5).

UPPER HAMSTRING PAIN

See: Upper leg (p. 90).

BOWLER'S BACK

Same stress fracture as Gymnast's
Back C.
See: Cricket (Chapter 5).

BUTTOCK BURSA PAIN

DIAGNOSIS:
(a) Lie on stomach; pain in buttock
muscles when straight leg raised

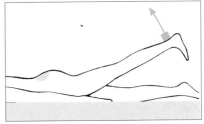

(b) Lying on front, raise leg and block at
position shown; pain at top of buttock.

CAUSE:
Overwork makes fluid-filled sac (bursa)
under buttock muscle sore.

TREATMENT:
Self: Rest.
Medical: Interferential. Laser, ultrasound.
Cortisone injection. Check circulation.

TRAINING:
Continue as usual; pain harmless, but
running may flare it. Avoid stiff-kneed
running style, sprints, hill-running,
swinging straightened leg. Some martial
arts sports drills cause pains.

Low back pain

Since there are many causes of low back pain, medical advice should be sought, especially for teenage back problems. Fractures have not been covered.

MECHANICAL PROBLEMS

DIAGNOSIS:
Pain is produced in back or leg by some of the following: coughing, sneezing, sitting, standing from sitting position, bending forward/backward/to one side, raising straight leg when lying flat on back.

CAUSE:
Damaged disc or facet joint in spine.

TREATMENT:
Rest will help, but seek medical advice, especially for teenagers. Treatment may vary, even for same person on different occasions, so the following are only guidelines:
Self:
• Bedrest.
• Stretching: Hang from arms 5-10 minutes (resting when necessary); some portable machines support feet in straps, while body hangs upside down.
• Sustained self-manipulation: Lie with pain free side on edge of bed, keep shoulders flat on bed, twist pelvis and leg on painful side up and over other leg to hang over edge, hold 15-20 minutes.
Medical: Some guidelines on medical treatment:
• Sudden pain (may leave person unable to move): Painkillers, rest, manipulation, epidural injection.

• Slow onset of pain (gradual stiffening after gardening or long exercise): Painkillers, rest, traction, epidural injection, support corset.
• Sciatica (pain felt in leg, even down to foot, from disc pressing on spinal nerve): Painkillers, rest, traction, epidural injection, support corset.
• Sciatica with weak muscles (muscles weak due to nerve damage): Painkillers, bed rest, epidural injection, check no diabetes or cause other than disc, support corset.
• Night pain (burning leg pain severe enough to wake at night – not just pain when turning over in bed): Rest; painkillers; epidural injection; support corset.
• Shooting pain (down leg): Epidural injection; manipulation; not traction.
• Pains worse with extension. May be "collar stud" disc, but check facet joint for spondylolysis or spondylolisthesis, especially in teenagers.

NOTE
If treatment is unsuccessful, surgery may be required.

PROBLEM BACKS

Problem backs can be pigeonholed into two main but overlapping categories, which we call Group A and Group B for easy reference. By following the tips on the next few pages, you can find out which type of back shape you have and then how to adjust your posture in order to avoid back pain.

CORRECTING YOUR POSTURE

GROUP A
Rounded Back (1, 2, 3)
The pain is worse bending over, sitting, driving and especially getting out of a chair when the back feels a little stuck. Feels better when lying face down and arching backward. More low back hollow is required. Let your weight come forward towards the balls of the feet.

GROUP B
Hollowed (Sway) Back (1, 2, 3)
Applies to those whose pain is worse standing relaxed, leaning backward, lying face down, eased by half-sitting on desk, or stool. Less low back hollow is required, more flattening of pelvis. Stand with your weight back, towards heels.

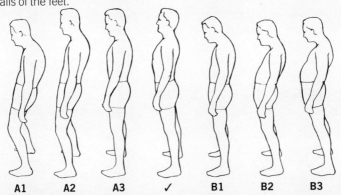

A1   A2   A3   ✓   B1   B2   B3

A1 Straighten knees, placing weight on balls of feet to allow hollow in small of back. Straighten upper back, standing tall. Draw back head on shoulders.

A2 Allow hollow in small of back, but flatten stomach muscles. Stand tall through upper spine; straighten head and shoulders.

A3 Too straight; let hollow come into small of back – stand with weight on balls of feet.

✓ The **neutral position** has tolerance, and is the ideal posture. Stand with weight balanced over the middle of both feet, with slight hollow in the low back, stomach muscles gently tightened and upper back straightened. Draw chin and head back, not up. Don't just draw your shoulders back like a sergeant major.

B1 Stand taller through upper back; straighten round back and straighten head and neck.

B2 Flatten stomach to support back.

B3 Tilt pelvis forward to flatten lower back, shift weight towards the heels

Bending

Most people have experienced pain or twinges in the back when bending and lifting. This could be when picking up a box of groceries or brushing their teeth. It could be leaning in to pull something out of the car or adjusting a sail on a boat. The trick is to use the proper neutral back position, bend your knees and stick your bottom out.

Use neutral position. Squat lower in between legs. Do not lose neutral position by flattening or rounding back. Half bends when brushing teeth, for example, should also be done this way.

Tips for getting back to normal.

GROUP A AND B

• Use neutral position all the time – day in, day out – especially when carrying, leaning or bending over.
• Sitting: Sit, with buttocks as far back in chair (preferably one with straight back) as possible. Knees should be same height as, or lower than, hips. Don't sit in low chairs or on low steps, because getting up can be difficult.
• Getting up from lying position: Turn on to side, bend knees and slide feet off bed onto floor. Then sit up sideways.
• Standing from sitting position: Move buttocks to front part of chair or bed, keep neutral position. Turn sideways and draw both feet (one behind the other) back under knees. Then stand up using the neutral position. Push with hands if possible for more support; choose chairs with arms.

GROUP A

• Sitting: Place pillows in small of back. Hollow back if slumping. If in soft deep sofa, or in office chair for a long day, sit forward, turn sideways and drop one knee to point towards floor. This will help to arch back. Condition is helped by 'kneel-on' chairs.
• Sleep on firm mattress or with board underneath mattress. Try sleeping face down.

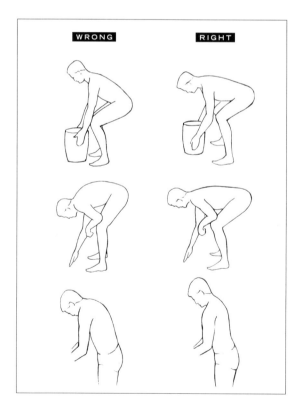

GROUP B

- Sitting: Allow to slump. No pillows in back. Not helped by 'kneel-on' chairs.
- Standing: Helped by standing with one foot supported 6-8 in. (15-20 cm.) off ground using a box, chair strut or bar rail
- Sleep on softer mattress. Lie in any position that is comfortable. With sciatica down front of leg and shin, try placing pillow underneath knees when lying on back or underneath hips when lying on front.

Sports training with back problems
Weight training is designed for specific muscle groups. If and when you have to use your back to help with lifting, then the muscles you are working on have become tired, so stop.

- Weight training must be done with a neutral back – as soon as this position is threatened by tiredness, stop.
- Use counterbalanced weight machines so that the back may be supported sitting or lying down – these are much better than free weights.

Sit-ups for back
GROUP A AND B
- Lie on back, knees bent, feet flat on ground. Curl head and shoulders towards belly button. Hold or rock gently.
GROUP A
- Raise both legs straight off floor. Hold about 6 in. (15 cm.) above floor. Use Rule of 7 (p. 131).
GROUP B
- Lie on back, bend knees and hips to lift feet off floor. Straighten knees – hold neutral back. Lower straight legs until

want to arch back. Stop, and move legs towards head until back is comfortable; hold as long as can. Bend knees and hips to come down.

There are many other exercises for backs that may be found in specialist books. Always bear in mind that exercises which force the back towards its problem position i.e. bent forward for Group A or backward for Group B, may accentuate the trouble.

AVOID
- Heavy weights that cannot be lifted easily. Use lighter weights instead, increasing repetitions.
- Working too fast. Always maintain neutral position.
- Squats with weights.
- Step-ups.
- Lifting weights from floor.
- Any weight training that does not keep body supported lying down or that moves it away from vertical position, e.g., upright rowing.
- Doing anything that hurts.

General fitness training
DO
- Bicycle, but remember to sit upright. If you have drop handlebars, reverse them.
- Swim, find most comfortable stroke – Group A, freestyle; Group B, probably backstroke. Don't dive in; use steps to climb out.
- Stairmaster machine.
- Patter, then skipping routine (p. 129).
- When above can be done with no pain, follow Achilles top ladder (p. 142).

Exercises

WARNING

While one part is injured, try to keep other areas fit. Do not try to work through pain. Apply power just until discomfort starts; hold, but go no further.

CALVES:

Heels: Stand on balls of feet on edge of step, facing upstairs. Dropping heels as low as possible, rise to tiptoe and then lower heels slowly.

QUADRICEPS:

• Bicycle: Use low resistance with fast pedal rate – build to high resistance.
• Wall exercise: Standing with back straight against wall, slide down so thighs are at about 100° angle to floor; hold 7 seconds, rest 7 seconds, for 3 minutes. Do not go lower than 90° angle. Try one leg at a time.
• Sit in chair with back supported; put carrier bag or basket over foot with bags of sugar inside to make up weight. Slowly lift up so leg is straight, counting 7 seconds, then lower leg, again taking 7 seconds. Repeat 8-10 times.
• Use quadriceps machine if available.
• Sit on table; hook heel over appropriate ankle. Push away with back foot, pull back with front foot.

HAMSTRING:

• Standing, hook heel under chair; pull towards bottom (put a weight on chair). Alter angle of knee when starting exercise, from nearly straight to fully bent. Hold 7 seconds as hard as possible, relax 7 seconds, for 2-3 minutes.
• Use hamstring training machine if available. Tie a theraband or elastic loop such as inner tube of a bicycle around

ankle and fixed object; bend knee and foot towards bottom against the stretch of the rubber.

BUTTOCKS:

Sit on floor with legs straight out. "Walk" forward on your bottom, then backward for 2 minutes.

STOMACH MUSCLES:

See: Sit-ups for backs (p. 81).

NOTE

Do not do these exercises if they cause pain.

BACK MUSCLES:

• Swallows: Lie on stomach on floor, hands behind head, raise shoulders from floor. If able, also raise feet off floor at same time. Hold 10 seconds, relax 10 seconds, for 2-3 minutes.
• Use back extension machine in gymnasium.

SHOULDERS:

• Lie on back on floor; hold book (or weights) in each hand. With arms outstretched (90° angle to chest), raise both arms so books touch over chest.
• press-ups: Hold onto bar or tree branch above head. Pull body up to touch bar with chin only as far as possible, using both overhand and underhand grip to exercise different muscles. Repeat as often as comfortable.
• Dips: Stand between bars or chairbacks. Support body weight on hands on bars/chairs. Drop elbows to 90° angle, then raise to straighten arms. Repeat as often as comfortable.
• Press-ups: Lie face down on floor, hands on floor by shoulders. Keep body straight, maintaining neutral position; push shoulders up to arms' length. Drop

elbows to right angles, then push straight again. Repeat as often as comfortable. If you are in pain or not strong enough, press up first from table, later from chair, later kneeling on floor, later full push-up.

WARNING

Any doubts, failure to progress, constant pain that does not change with movement, or feeling unwell, consult doctor.

MUSCLE CRAMP OR SPASM

CAUSE:
Cramp/spasm usually caused by a mechanical problem.

TREATMENT:
Self: Rest. Painkillers. Hot-water bottle.
Medical: Treat mechanical problem. Massage. Interferential. Laser, ultrasound.

LIGAMENT STRAINS IN BACK (Cocktail party back)

DIAGNOSIS:
Back muscles are stiff and sore first thing in morning but ease with movement until you do too much. Sitting or standing for long periods produces dull backache relieved by shifting and moving around. All back movements have full range, but all may hurt. Straight leg raise is pain free, though may feel stiff.

CAUSE:
May follow mechanical problems but can be due to bad posture, especially during pregnancy and before menstrual period.

TREATMENT:
Self: Maintain neutral position; do not slouch, especially when resting. This is a safe back condition, so sports may be played; back will be trouble free during exercise, but will ache and feel weak afterward. May need to squat down. Take NSAIDs.
Medical: NSAIDs. Laser, ultrasound. Sugar injections into ligaments to strengthen them (prolotherapy).

HIP AND PELVIS

A complicated area, linking the legs to the body via the ball-and-socket hip joints, the hip stabilizer muscles and then a ring – the pelvis – which joins the sacroiliac joints to the spine. When this ring is disturbed the damage occurs at more than one place, so injuries are often complicated. The hip is a strong joint with a wide range of movements. Unfortunately, stretching exercises to maintain this movement are often ignored: compare the somewhat limited movement of the average runner with that of a dancer, gymnast or karate exponent. Injuries to the sacroiliac joint and the mid back can often cause pain in this area.

MEDICAL NOTE

Stress fractures can occur in the pelvis. These invariably get worse with activity, and feel better at rest. If pains do not fit any diagnostic pattern, bone scan or x-ray required. Stress fractures may occur in sacrum, ischiopubic ramus, and femoral neck.

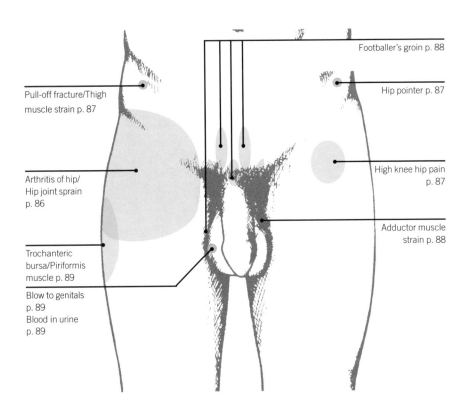

Footballer's groin p. 88

Hip pointer p. 87

Pull-off fracture/Thigh muscle strain p. 87

High knee hip pain p. 87

Arthritis of hip/ Hip joint sprain p. 86

Adductor muscle strain p. 88

Trochanteric bursa/Piriformis muscle p. 89

Blow to genitals p. 89
Blood in urine p. 89

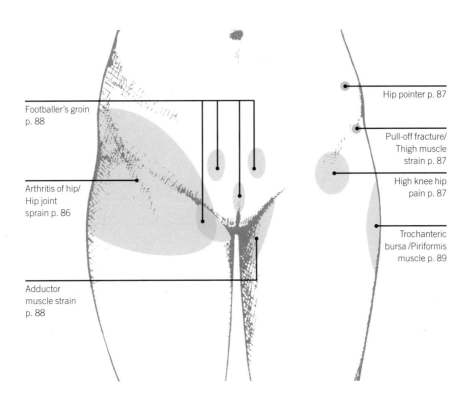

Footballer's groin
p. 88

Arthritis of hip/
Hip joint
sprain p. 86

Adductor
muscle strain
p. 88

Hip pointer p. 87

Pull-off fracture/
Thigh muscle
strain p. 87

High knee hip
pain p. 87

Trochanteric
bursa /Piriformis
muscle p. 89

ARTHRITIS OF HIP/HIP JOINT SPRAIN (Capsulitis)

DIAGNOSIS:

Lie on back so that leg can be moved as shown in diagrams. Small movements may not hurt but all will be painful at final or extended range. Pain may be felt in knee.

CAUSE:

Wear and tear on joint, or hip sprain; the latter takes up to 3 weeks to get better. Arthritis persists after sprain healed. Usually occurs late thirties onward, but sometimes at very early age.

TREATMENT:

Self: Always rest and seek medical help for children. NSAIDs. Warm baths. Restrict range of movement of hip. Rest. *Medical:* Rest. NSAIDs. Shortwave diathermy. Interferential. Cortisone injection. Surgery: replacement hip.

TRAINING:

Warm bath before training may help. Normal general fitness routine; pattering, rowing, bike, but not breaststroke in swimming. Do not overstretch joint in any direction, e.g. keep stride length short.

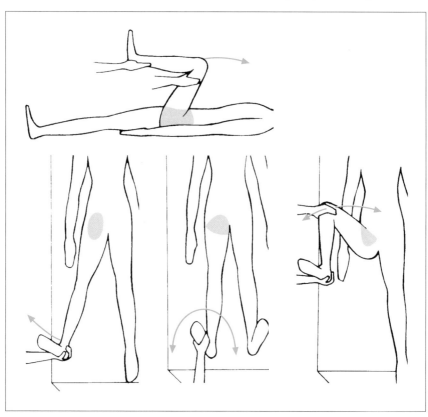

Pattering footwork essential for twisting sports. May signal end of sports involving running or twisting. Play doubles tennis rather than squash or racquetball. See: Golf (Chapter 5). Home and Workplace (p. 156).

HIGH KNEE HIP PAIN (Psoas bursa)

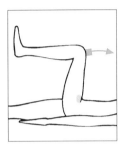

DIAGNOSIS:
Lie on back, leg raised and bent as in diagram. Block movement towards body; pain confirmed at hip joint.

CAUSE:
Overuse makes bursa (or fluid-filled sac) under muscle that bends hip sore. Example: sudden increase in sprint training, hill-running, running or speed skating (with upper body leaning forward). Not a muscle tear.

TREATMENT:
Self: Rest. Stretching exercise 8.
Medical: Laser, ultrasound. Cortisone injection.

TRAINING:
Normal general fitness routine, but avoid sprints, hill-running, squat thrusts. See: Hockey (field), Skating, Track and Field Athletics (Chapter 5).

HIP POINTER/HIP CONTUSION

DIAGNOSIS:
Bruising on front, top of hipbone. Thigh will not move forward.

CAUSE:
Blow to or fall onto hipbone. Full-length dive in baseball, heavy tackle in football.

TREATMENT:
Self: RICE. If in pain, consult doctor.
Medical: Laser, ultrasound. Interferential. Possibly haematoma.

TRAINING:
Normal general fitness routine, but avoid sprints, hill-running, squat thrusts.

PULL-OFF FRACTURE/THIGH MUSCLE STRAIN

DIAGNOSIS:
Area hurts to touch; may show bruise or puffy swelling.

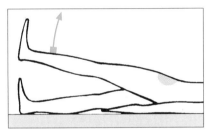

Lie on back and block upward movement of leg as in diagram; pain confirmed at hip joint. Pull-off mainly occurs in adolescents; adults can damage same area where tendon goes into bone.

CAUSE:
Muscle pulls away from bone due to very sudden contraction. Usually occurs in teenagers, especially in kicking sports, or sudden sprints.

TREATMENT:
Self: Rest 6-8 weeks.
Medical: Controlled loading of muscle

using TENS or interferential. Note muscle can produce myositis ossificans. Rest 6-8 weeks.

TRAINING:
Fitness – Hamstring ladders; low gears on bike.
Strength – Heels (see p. 140, step 6), upper body work; quads ladder.
Stretch – All stretching exercises but stop at onset of pain with exercises 8, 10, 12.
See: Badminton/Skating/Hockey (Chapter 5).

FOOTBALLER'S GROIN
(Osteitis pubis symphysis, Conjoined tendon)

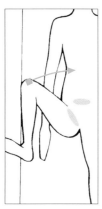

DIAGNOSIS:
• As for Adductor muscle strain (below), but may produce low stomach pain later.
• Hurts in middle of pubis.
• Turning, even turning over in bed, may be painful in low stomach and groin.
• Sit-ups may hurt.
• Kicking, sprinting may hurt.
• Lie on back. Block movement of leg towards body as shown in diagram. Pain confirmed in groin.

CAUSE:
Ligament joining pelvic bones in front becomes loose. May appear during pregnancy or after giving birth. Thought to be due to overloading one leg more than other as in repeated kicking favouring one foot, high hurdles (leading with the same leg), or hard side step and backing off in front of opponents while twisting from side to side (as midfielders in soccer).

TREATMENT:
Self: May rest or play within pain, takes months to heal. Seek medical advice.
Medical: Rest. Treat accompanying adductor muscle. Flamingo x-ray or scan to exclude bone damage. Early stage of problem may be conjoined tendon from abdominal muscles or even small crypt hernia (tender external ring). Surgery may be treatment of choice.

TRAINING:
Achilles ladders, taken slowly, then knee ladder.
See: Basketball, Soccer, Football, Hockey (field), Rugby (Chapter 5).

ADDUCTOR MUSCLE STRAIN

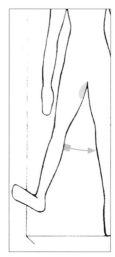

DIAGNOSIS:
• Lying down, block leg movement inward at knee as shown. Pain confirmed in groin.
• May be tender over bone in groin or just off/on tendon. Check for Footballer's groin immediately, may be difficult. Consult doctor.

CAUSE:

Adductor muscles pull thighs and knees together, so strain may occur when sidestepping or skipping sideways. Sprinting acceleration, with knees turned in and feet out, may cause strain; also hill-running, when knees and feet are turned out to get shorter stride going uphill, particularly when tired and in mud.

TREATMENT:

Self: RICE. Cross-frictional massage. Stretching exercises 4, 9, 10, 12; if no improvement, see Footballer's groin. *Medical:* Laser, ultrasound. Frictional massage. Cortisone injection.

TRAINING:

Achilles ladders, then knee ladders. See: Track and Field Athletics, Fencing, Badminton, Football (Rugby and American) (Chapter 5).

TROCHANTERIC BURSA/PIRIFORMIS

DIAGNOSIS:

Hurts to press outside of bony point of hip. Movements for arthritis diagnosis do not hurt.

Lie on side on floor, painful hip on top, raise and block straight leg sideways;

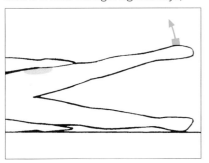

pain confirmed. Pain near same area at back on bony knob may be a muscle problem of the piriformis.

CAUSE:

Sitting one leg crossed over other for a long time in the office. Direct blow (squash player slamming into wall) or severe exertion (running extra half hour one day) irritates bursa, or fluid-filled sac; extra fluid inflames area and any movement maintains inflammation.

TREATMENT:

Self: RICE. NSAIDs. Avoid sitting with legs crossed at knees; avoid disco dancing. *Medical:* Laser, ultrasound. Interferential. Cortisone injection. Stretch ileo-tibial band.

TRAINING:

Continue as usual, unless painful.

BLOW TO GENITALS

TREATMENT:

Prevent by wearing protective cup. *Self:* Painkillers (men: elevate by wearing support). If blood appears in urine, seek medical advice at once. See: Water skiing (Chapter 5).

BLOOD IN URINE

Seek medical advice. (May not be serious if it follows exercise.)

UPPER LEG

The hamstring is at risk in sports where players stop and start suddenly, especially when sprinting. It crosses both knee and hip joints, and at times one end of the muscle is tightening while the other is relaxing. Picture the whiplash effect going through the muscle at that moment! That is why it is important to build up this coordination as part of the treatment, before testing an injured leg in competition. Sometimes damage to the hamstring may occur because the muscle is weak, but it can also occur because it is stronger than the other leg and is therefore overcompensating. There should also be a balance between the hamstring on the back of the leg and the powerful quadriceps on the front.

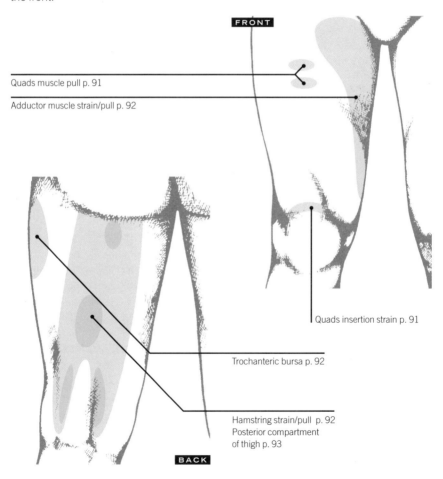

FRONT

Quads muscle pull p. 91

Adductor muscle strain/pull p. 92

Quads insertion strain p. 91

Trochanteric bursa p. 92

Hamstring strain/pull p. 92
Posterior compartment
of thigh p. 93

BACK

QUADS INSERTION STRAIN

DIAGNOSIS:
Pain just above and on top of edge of kneecap. Treat as for Quads muscle pull. See: Quads expansion (p. 99).

CAUSE:
Overuse injury, particularly from squats, hill-running, etc. Onset more gradual than quads pull, but the same muscle, spreading out over kneecap and its tendons, is involved.

TREATMENT:
Self: RICE. Play is usually still possible, but injury will persist. Stretching exercises 8, 10.
Medical: Cross-frictional massage. Laser, ultrasound. Cortisone injection.

TRAINING:
Continue as usual, but avoid squats, especially with weights, squat thrusts, step-ups and hill-running. Use Quads ladder for strength training.

QUADS MUSCLE PULL

DIAGNOSIS:
Front of upper leg hurts to touch. May produce bruise around knee. Soreness when going upstairs, up hills, doing squats, kicking.

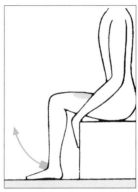

Sitting, block upward movement of leg; pain confirmed.

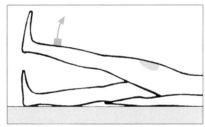

Lying on back, block upward movement of leg at point indicated; pain confirmed.

CAUSE:
Usually central muscle tear, causing damage in 2 areas about 2 in. (50 mm.) apart. Sometimes muscle tears away from kneecap, producing lump in thigh, especially if kick is blocked. Treatment:
Self: RICE. Stretching exercises 8, 10. Muscle-taping.
Medical: Laser, ultrasound. Frictional massage, isokinetics. Rarely surgery.

Quads ladder.
See: Badminton, Cycling, Gymnastics, Hockey (field), Rugby, Skating, Skiing, Soccer, Squash, Weight lifting (Chapter 5).

ADDUCTOR MUSCLE STRAIN/PULL

DIAGNOSIS:
Hurts to touch. Perhaps bruise over tender spot and/or inside of knee.
See: Hip and pelvis – Adductor muscle strain.

CAUSE:
See: Hip and pelvis – Adductor muscle strain.

TREATMENT:
Self: See: Hip and pelvis. Also strap for training. Stretching exercises 4, 9 mainly; also 10, 12.
Medical: Laser, ultrasound. Frictional massage.

TRAINING:
General muscle ladder to stage 5; combine with Achilles ladder to stage 8; then Knee ladder to stage 5; then Achilles ladder stages 9-12.
See: Badminton, Soccer (Chapter 5).

Back upper leg

TROCHANTERIC BURSA

See: Hip and pelvis.

HAMSTRING STRAIN/PULL

DIAGNOSIS:
• Tender to touch; tenderness may seem to move around 2-3 different areas during healing.
• May show bruise over tender area and/or behind knee; heals faster than when no bruise.
• Leaning backward and running hands down either side does not hurt.
• Bending to touch toes hurts tender area.

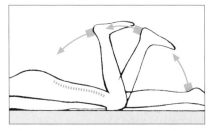

Lying on front, block leg movements as shown in diagram; pain down back of thigh.

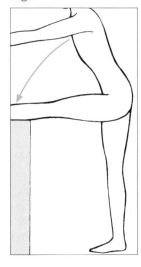

Standing in position in diagram, bend down towards leg; pain down back of thigh. Pain here can be deceptive. Might not be muscle problem but sciatica, but hamstring has no

accompanying back pain.
See: Low back (p. 78).

CAUSE:

Movement of hip and knee out of natural phase, so muscle tears, especially if hamstring taut with no reserve elasticity. Can result from insufficient warming up; common in explosive events involving sprinting. Do not force hurdle stretch exercise as this may produce injury where hamstring attaches to the bone you sit on! Always relax into stretch and breathe out. Do not force.

TREATMENT:

Self: RICE. Patience required as will recur if not fully healed.

Medical: Deep friction and effluage, massages. Laser, ultrasound. Check leg length. Isokinetics may show up muscle imbalance. Check sciatic nerve, primary posterolateral disc, sacroiliac joint and pelvic alignment. If there is pain at the ischeal tuberosity, bone scan may be positive. Injection. Surgery.

TRAINING:

General muscle ladder stages 1-6, combined with Hamstring ladders. Bottom ladder provides fitness, top ladder muscle re-education, which gradually becomes sprint-type fitness.

POSTERIOR COMPARTMENT OF THIGH

In rare cases hamstring muscles are held too tightly by muscle sheathes that cut down blood supply to muscle.

DIAGNOSIS:

Condition appears with running over longer distances at speed. Usually effects high-class athletes. Worse on hard ground.

TREATMENT:

Self: RICE. Elevation more important than compression.

Medical: Establish diagnosis. Exclude hamstring, sciatica, sacroiliac joint, stress fracture, hamstring and piriformis syndrome. Surgery.

TRAINING:

Train on softer ground; reduce speed and mileage.

KNEE

This is the most injury-prone of all the joints; it is especially susceptible to falls and twists. Severe damage may occur in flat-out competition, but problems are often caused in training, where the knee is overused and abused in unbalanced and badly planned sessions. The anatomy of the individual knee may also be at fault, and this may be corrected by altering the balance of the foot. Many training schedules combine strength, endurance and stamina, but these can be broken down into component parts if overuse injuries occur.

Take cycling, for example. Road race cyclists consistently rate in the top fitness group. Why not, therefore, spend two days of your week on a bicycle to take the impact off your knees? You would reach the same standards of fitness, with less wear and tear on your knees. This is particularly true of anyone training for a marathon, whether he or she is just taking part or running to win.

WARNING

This section is designed not only to help you understand your injury but also to train with it once it has been diagnosed. Do not rely on self-diagnosis. This is a diagnostic minefield even for doctors, so consult an expert when you suffer knee pain.

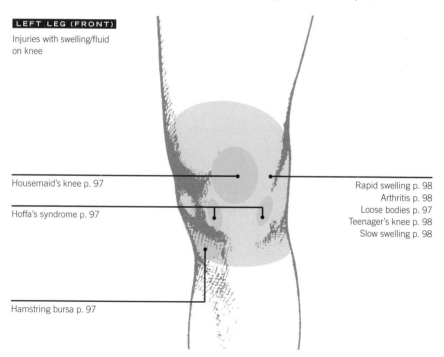

LEFT LEG (FRONT)
Injuries with swelling/fluid on knee

Housemaid's knee p. 97

Hoffa's syndrome p. 97

Hamstring bursa p. 97

Rapid swelling p. 98
Arthritis p. 98
Loose bodies p. 97
Teenager's knee p. 98
Slow swelling p. 98

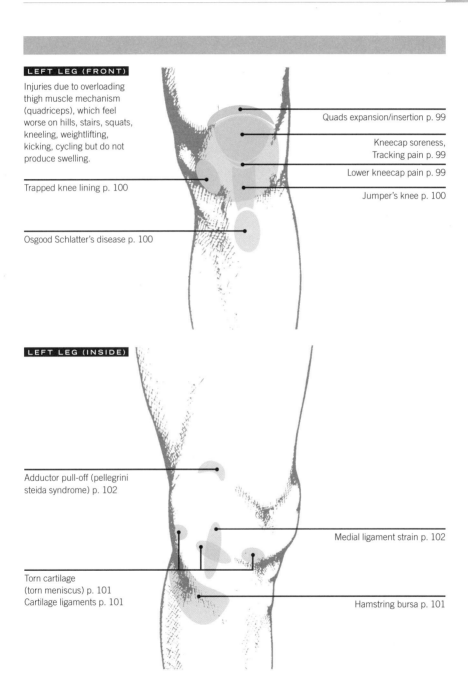

LEFT LEG (FRONT)

Injuries due to overloading thigh muscle mechanism (quadriceps), which feel worse on hills, stairs, squats, kneeling, weightlifting, kicking, cycling but do not produce swelling.

Quads expansion/insertion p. 99

Kneecap soreness, Tracking pain p. 99

Lower kneecap pain p. 99

Trapped knee lining p. 100

Jumper's knee p. 100

Osgood Schlatter's disease p. 100

LEFT LEG (INSIDE)

Adductor pull-off (pellegrini steida syndrome) p. 102

Medial ligament strain p. 102

Torn cartilage (torn meniscus) p. 101
Cartilage ligaments p. 101

Hamstring bursa p. 101

KNEE

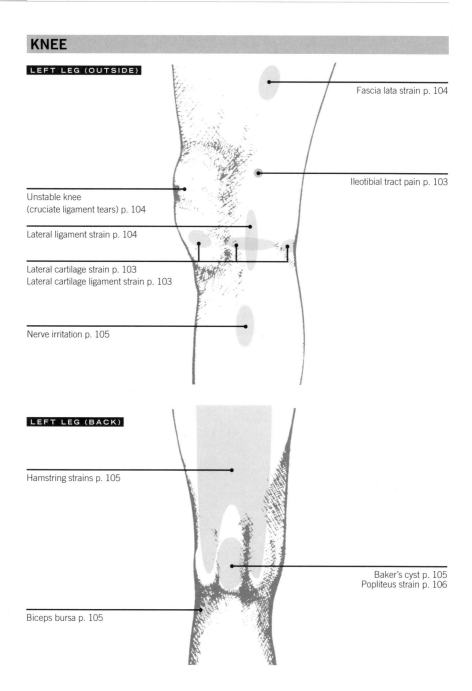

LEFT LEG (OUTSIDE)

Fascia lata strain p. 104

Ileotibial tract pain p. 103

Unstable knee
(cruciate ligament tears) p. 104

Lateral ligament strain p. 104

Lateral cartilage strain p. 103
Lateral cartilage ligament strain p. 103

Nerve irritation p. 105

LEFT LEG (BACK)

Hamstring strains p. 105

Baker's cyst p. 105
Popliteus strain p. 106

Biceps bursa p. 105

Swelling/Fluid on knee

HOUSEMAID'S KNEE
(Prepatellar bursa)

DIAGNOSIS:
May or may not be tender. Fluid under skin but outside knee joint.

CAUSE:
Too much kneeling; direct blow over kneecap.

TREATMENT:
Self: Avoid kneeling. RICE. Maintain compression until advised otherwise. NSAIDs.
Medical: Leave alone. Do nothing. Occasionally drain off fluid. Cortisone injection. NSAIDs.

TRAINING:
Normal general fitness routine. See: Canoeing, Shooting (Chapter 5), Home and Workplace (p. 156).

HOFFA'S SYNDROME

DIAGNOSIS:
Hollows either side of knee joint appear swollen (this is fat, not fluid); tender to press.

CAUSE:
Overuse, usually in long-distance runners, especially at end of run, or joggers who increase mileage too suddenly. Hill-running, particularly downhill, can bring it on.

TREATMENT:
Self: RICE. NSAIDs. Be sure shoes have thick, shock-absorbent soles.
Medical: Laser, ultrasound. Cortisone injection. Can be associated with tracking problems (knock-knees, pronated feet).

TRAINING:
Reduce mileage. Run on grass if possible. Avoid downhill runs.

HAMSTRING BURSA
(Semimembranosus bursa)

DIAGNOSIS:
Inside and lower part of knee tender to touch.

CAUSE:
Overuse of hamstrings. Especially if running style is not "bounding" but more of a shuffle. Worse if the foot turns out. Occasionally occurs when compensating for another knee injury.

TREATMENT:
Self: RICE. NSAIDs.
Medical: Laser, ultrasound. Frictional massage. Cortisone injection.

TRAINING:
Continue as usual, but avoid bending knee rapidly as in cycling or sprinting. Alter running style, especially if knees splay outward.

LOOSE BODIES

DIAGNOSIS:
Knee may lock or stick. May be swelling.

CAUSE:
Loose fragments of cartilage or bone within knee.

TREATMENT:
Self: RICE. NSAIDs.
Medical: X-ray. MRI. Arthroscope. Surgery.

TRAINING:
Rest. Use Knee ladder under medical supervision.

TEENAGER'S KNEE
(Osteochondritis dissecans)

DIAGNOSIS:
Doctors can see loose bodies on x-ray, CT scan or MRI, doctor can see injury and assess whether loose bodies are present.

CAUSE:
Small piece of bone and cartilage separates and can form loose body in knee joint. More common in boys.

TREATMENT:
Self: RICE. NSAIDs.
Medical: Allow to heal by itself, if no loose body. Surgery.

TRAINING:
Rest. Knee ladder under medical supervision.

ARTHRITIS

DIAGNOSIS:
Knee may be painful at rest, worse with movement. Fully straightening and fully bending hurts. May cause swelling.

CAUSE:
As cartilage wears down, kneebones roughen from grating together. May follow surgical removal of meniscus.

TREATMENT:
Self: Rest. NSAIDs. Warm bath.
Medical: NSAIDs. Shortwave diathermy. Cortisone injection. Knee brace, quads muscle exercises. Orthotics. Surgery.

TRAINING:
Do not over-exercise joint; space out training with rest intervals. Avoid impact in training. Although it is safe to be active, do not run or jump; instead swim, cycle or row. May end competitive sports/very active games.

RAPID SWELLING (within 2-4 hours)

DIAGNOSIS:
Swelling occurs within 2-4 hours. Blood in joint. Usually anterior cruciate ligament.

TREATMENT:
Self: RICE; crutches maintain compression until advised otherwise. Seek medical advice within 2-4 days – at latest within 14 days. NSAIDs.
Medical: Drain fluid. Fat globules in blood indicate fracture present. MRI. Physiotherapy and rehabilitation. Surgery. Check fractured tibia plateau, dislocated patella, posterior cruciate ligament. Peripheral meniscal tear.

TRAINING:
To be combined with specific rehabilitation from physiotherapist/ trainer. Heels. Quads ladder. Sit-ups. Upper body strength. Knee ladder. See: Badminton, Skiing (Chapter 5).

SLOW SWELLING (from 6-24 hours)

DIAGNOSIS:
Swelling occurs from 6-24 hours.

CAUSE:
Varied – may be sprained, or as serious as torn cartilage.

TREATMENT:

Self: RICE; maintain ice and compression over 7-4 days, may settle by itself. NSAIDs.

Medical: Aspirate to exclude crystals, infection or blood. If clear yellow fluid, await events. Sticking, catching history – check meniscus or loose body. MRI.

TRAINING:

See Rapid swelling, above.

Injuries due to overloading thigh muscle mechanism

QUADS EXPANSION/INSERTION

DIAGNOSIS:

Pain at top of kneecap.

CAUSE:

Overload of quads muscles.

TREATMENT:

Self: RICE. Frictional massage.

Medical: Deep friction massage. Laser, ultrasound. Cortisone injection. Stretch 8.

TRAINING:

Quads ladder. Avoid strenuous bent knees exercise, e.g., climbing hills, squats, step-ups, squat thrusts, weights. See: Badminton, Cycling, Gymnastics, Hockey (field), Rugby, Skating, Skiing, Squash, Weight lifting (Chapter 5).

KNEECAP SORENESS/TRACKING PAIN

DIAGNOSIS:

Pain on either or both sides of kneecap. Difficult to bend knee, worse when sitting. More common in women.

CAUSE:

Inflammation at back of kneecap. Caused by a tracking problem (faulty alignment of kneecap in groove of thighbone); also overloading quadriceps muscles (weights, hill-running, stairs, etc.) will produce more pressure on badly tracking kneecap.

TREATMENT:

Self: Rest. Lie on floor with light – 5 lb. (2 kg.) – weight on ankle of sore leg; place cushion under knee and extend leg from 20° to straight; gradually build up weight, but not degree of bend. Stand tall on one leg if you can; keeping buttocks tight, lock knee of that leg straight. Now slowly bend your knee, keeping knee vertically above big and second toes. Hold for a count of 7 seconds, then straighten leg again. Relax buttocks. Repeat.

Medical: Work on vastus medialis. McConnell strapping. Patella brace, orthotics for overpronation. Posterior tibialis strength. Surgery.

TRAINING:

Quads ladder. Avoid strenuous bent knee exercise such as climbing hills, squats, step-ups, squat thrusts, weights. Raise saddle on bike to straighten knee. See: Badminton, Cycling, Gymnastics, Hockey (field), Rowing, Rugby, Skating, Skiing, Squash, Weight lifting (Chapter 5).

LOWER KNEECAP PAIN
(Lower patella pole)

DIAGNOSIS:

Lower end of kneecap tender to touch; worse with stairs, squats, jumping, kicking.

CAUSE:
Overload, often by athletes who land or take off on one leg; also possible both legs.

TREATMENT:
Self: Deep friction massage.
Medical: Deep friction massage. Laser, ultrasound. Cortisone injection. Children may have growing area. (Sindig Larson Johansson.)

TRAINING:
Quads ladder. Avoid strenuous bent knee exercise such as climbing hills, squats, step-ups, squat thrusts, weights.
See: Badminton, Cricket, Cycling, Gymnastics, Hockey (field), Rugby, Skating, Skiing, Squash, Swimming, Weightlifting (Chapter 5).

TRAPPED KNEE LINING (Synovium)

DIAGNOSIS:
Pain either side of kneecap. Some movements pain free. Hurts to run, especially hill-running.

CAUSE:
Kneecap rubbing against thighbone.

TREATMENT:
Self: Rest.
Medical: Cortisone injection. Frictional massage. Orthotics, patellar brace. Surgery if plica is involved.

TRAINING:
Quads ladder. Avoid strenuous bent knee exercise such as climbing hills, squats, step-ups, squat thrusts, weights. Work on heels, Patter routine, Hamstring ladder.

JUMPER'S KNEE (Patella tendinitis)

DIAGNOSIS:
Thick tendon below kneecap tender to touch. Worse with stairs, squats, jumping, kicking.

CAUSE:
Overuse in jumping sports. Weights and explosive leg strength. Damaged tendon.

TREATMENT:
Self: RICE. Cross-frictional massage.
Medical: Rest. Laser, ultrasound. Cross-frictional massage for paratenon. Ultrasound scan or MRI scan may show degenerative cyst. Surgery.

TRAINING:
Quads ladder. Avoid strenuous bent knee exercise such as climbing hills, squats, step-ups, squat thrusts, weights.
See: Badminton, Squash, Basketball, Volleyball (Chapter 5).

OSGOOD SCHLATTER'S DISEASE

DIAGNOSIS:
Not really a disease but inflammation. Swelling and tenderness over knob below kneecap on shin. Occurs in growing children.

CAUSE:
Overuse; straining growing area where tendon attaches to bone. Does not occur when growth ceases but occasionally fragments may cause problems.

TREATMENT:
Self: Rest 4-12 weeks.
Medical: Controlled rest (within pain range). Surgery for residual fragments.

TRAINING:
Continue as usual, unless produces

pain. Quads ladder. Avoid strenuous bent knee exercise such as climbing hills, squats, step-ups, squat thrusts, weights, or a lot of kicking, until over about 16 years of age.
See: Badminton, Diving, Squash, Track and Field Athletics, Weightlifting, Rugby, Soccer (Chapter 5).

Pain on inside of knee

HAMSTRING BURSA

See p. 97.

TORN CARTILAGE/TORN MENISCUS

Medial cartilage is on inside of knee, lateral cartilage on outside.
DIAGNOSIS:
Gap between knee bones tender to press. Knee may be swollen and may stick, lock or click. Twisting and squatting may hurt.
CAUSE:
Forceful twisting tears or splits cartilage, the shock absorber in knee.
TREATMENT:
Self: RICE. Avoid twisting movements, support.
Medical: Await events. Parrot beak tear may settle by itself. Arthroscopy. Surgery.
TRAINING:
Quads ladder. Essential to maintain quads strength before and after operation. Rowing may be trouble-free type of exercise.

CARTILAGE LIGAMENTS

DIAGNOSIS:
Leg may not lock, but will catch with pain on certain knee movements. No swelling unless accompanied by other damage (i.e. torn cartilage). Tender to pressure over joint line or in hollows either side of knee, below kneecap.
CAUSE:
Ligaments are trapped between upper and lower legbone. Can be caused by running on camber or hump of road where, effectively, one leg is longer than the other; also running with lower legs

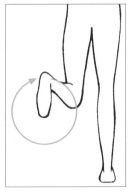

flailing or windmilling sideways (see diagram); also in hill-running, when tired legs mean lower knee lift and feet splaying out sideways; also sitting cross-legged or with feet tucked underneath chair or bottom.
TREATMENT:
Self: Rest. Massage over tender spot. Avoid hill-running, uneven surfaces, sitting cross-legged. Mount slopes zigzag fashion using short strides, foot planted directly below knee.
Medical: Frictional massage. Laser, ultrasound. Cortisone injection, correct foot if overpronating; orthotics.
TRAINING:
Continue as usual unless painful, but cut

down mileage, using several short circuits rather than one long one so you can return home if pain recurs; ensure knee lift is high to diminish rotation of lower leg. Avoid hills and rough ground until better. As kneeling or squatting may hurt, drop to one knee if you have to. Knee ladder for ball games.
See: Rugby, Sailing, Skiing, Soccer, Swimming (Chapter 5).

MEDIAL LIGAMENT STRAIN

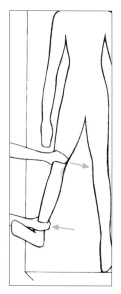

DIAGNOSIS: Pressing lower leg out sideways hurts. Tender to touch on inside of knee over joint line and just on either side over thighbone and on shinbone. Lying on back, legs apart as shown, leg is moved both out and in; pain confirmed on inside of knee. May bruise.

CAUSE: Severe wrenching of knee joint as lower leg goes out and sideways. May be severe enough to tear part or all of ligaments.

TREATMENT:
Self: RICE, especially compression, using support strapping or knee brace reaching 6 in. (15 cm.) above and below knee; too short a support is useless. Wear all day, every day, until Knee ladder started, then use in training and for first 6 weeks of competition.

WARNING
This treatment is sufficient if ligament not ruptured. If in doubt, see doctor within 10 days.
Medical: Rest. Hinged brace. Frictional massage. Laser, ultrasound. Surgery.

TRAINING:
As this ligament is vital to knee stability it must not be put at risk. Can take 3-4 months or longer to heal. Continue upper body work. Use Quads ladders without pattering. Knee ladder. All exercise to be done with knee support in place, also first 6 weeks of competition.
See: Skiing (Chapter 5).

ADDUCTOR PULL-OFF
(Pellegrini steida syndrome)

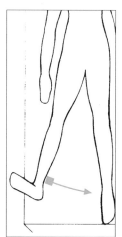

DIAGNOSIS: Highest knob of bone on inside of knee painful to pressure. Squeezing your fist or a tennis ball between knees causes pain over tender area. Lying on back, block inward movement of raised leg as shown; pain confirmed. Pain continues weeks after you think it should be better.

CAUSE:
Muscle or ligament on inside of thigh is pulled off when knee is wrenched; complicated by build-up of calcium and bone.

TREATMENT:
Self: RICE for 24 hours. Thorough rest required as exercise produces complication of new bone build-up; take medical advice before resuming even light exercise.
Medical: Rest. Surgery.

TRAINING:
General muscle ladder. Hamstring top ladder to step 9. Move to Knee ladder only if pain not getting worse for exercise or may re-flare injury.
See: Ball games and racquet sports (Chapter 5).

Pain on outside of knee

Most of these injuries are due to overuse strains but they occur more frequently with bowlegs, pigeon toes, running markedly on the outside of the foot, supination, flailing or windmilling the lower leg.

LATERAL CARTILAGE STRAIN

DIAGNOSIS:
If lump felt on the outside of knee joint comes and goes with knee movement, it is caused by swelling in the cartilage. See: Torn cartilage and Cartilage ligaments (p. 101). In case of cyst, leave alone if you have no trouble; if bothersome, may require surgery.

LATERAL CARTILAGE LIGAMENT STRAIN

DIAGNOSIS:
Does not lock knee; no swelling unless complicated by other knee problems. Twisting knee, full squat position and kneeling may hurt. Painful over gap between bones and/or in hollow on front of knee.

CAUSE:
Severe twist or continual pressure (even sitting cross-legged or with legs tucked under).

TREATMENT:
Self: RICE. Massage.
Medical: Rest. Cross-frictional massage. Laser, ultrasound. Orthotics.

TRAINING:
Continue as usual, but if too painful keep fit with rowing or freestyle swimming. Avoid deep knee bends, burpees. Avoid running on camber or hump of road. Flailing or windmilling lower leg should be avoided. When running, concentrate on lifting knee, shorter stride and smooth heel/toe action as foot lands. Avoid hill-running. Zigzag up slopes if you have to climb.
See: Soccer, Track and Field Athletics (pole vault) (Chapter 5).

ILEOTIBIAL TRACT PAIN

DIAGNOSIS:
When hand follows groove along outside of thigh, leg feels tender at bony knob on outside of knee. Hurts as knee bends this ileotibial tract from straight through 20-30°.

CAUSE:

Overuse in runners with awkward running styles.

TREATMENT:

Self: RICE. Frictional massage, reduce running. Consult coach.

Medical: Massage.Laser, ultrasound. Cortisone injection. Orthotics. Surgery.

TRAINING:

Runners may have to cross-train, using a different sport such as cycling or rowing. Running may have to be restricted to competitions only. Athletes in sports requiring quick changes of direction are rarely troubled. Avoid running on uneven, cambered or humped road where painful knee is out of balance with other leg.

FASCIA LATA STRAIN

DIAGNOSIS:

Pain in hollow or groove running down lower side of thigh to knee.

CAUSE:

Overuse in runners with awkward running styles.

TREATMENT:

Self: Rest. Use stretching exercise 6, but adapt with sore leg crossed behind other leg. RICE.

Medical: Rest. Laser, ultrasound. Orthotics.

TRAINING:

Avoid running downhill at speed and on camber or hump of road.

LATERAL LIGAMENT STRAIN

DIAGNOSIS:

Painful over gap between bones and over bones themselves. Hurts to force legs into bow-leg position.

CAUSE:

Wrenching knee sprains or tears ligament that holds knee in place.

TREATMENT:

Self: RICE. Strapping or knee brace; too short a support is useless. Wear all day, every day, until you can start on Knee ladder, then use brace for exercise and for first 6 weeks of competition.

WARNING

This treatment is sufficient if ligament not ruptured. If in doubt, see doctor within 10 days.

Medical: Rest. Hinged brace. NSAIDs. Laser, ultrasound. Cross-frictional massage. Surgery.

TRAINING:

No running. Swim, row, do bike routine, patter routine through to Knee ladder under medical direction. Maintain Quads ladder. Keep strapping support on throughout and for 6-8 weeks once back in action.

UNSTABLE KNEE
(Cruciate ligament tears)

DIAGNOSIS:

Only by doctor. If blood in knee or if, after major injury, knee still gives way even when apparently better. Check Medial ligament strain, p. 102 and Lateral ligament strain, above.

CAUSE:
Major wrenched knee.

TREATMENT:
Self: Support or strapping.
Medical: Physiotherapy. Braced knee support. Surgery.

TRAINING:
Under medical supervision. Closed chain exercises under medical control. Quads ladder. As most contact sports do not allow use of knee brace, you may have to change to new sport or have surgery.
See: Badminton, Skiing (Chapter 5).

NERVE IRRITATION

DIAGNOSIS:
Pain and/or numbness on outside of lower leg. Reproduced by pressing hollow just below lowest bony knob on outside of leg below knee.

CAUSE:
Damage, irritation to nerve after direct blow, awkward fall or running with bow legs. In extreme cases, even sitting with knees crossed!

TREATMENT:
Self: Painkillers. Will get better in 3 weeks or so if cause avoided. Avoid sitting cross-legged.
Medical: Irritation of the peroneal nerve around the fibular neck may mimic Anterior compartment syndrome (p. 110). Painkillers. Cortisone injection. Surgery.

TRAINING:
Orthotics or try lateral forefoot wedge. Continue as usual.
See: Track and Field Athletics (Chapter 5).

Pain on back of knee

HAMSTRING STRAINS

See: Back upper leg. May show up as bruises around knee. Will heal faster than same-sized tear that does not produce bruise.

BAKER'S CYST

DIAGNOSIS:
Lump in middle of back of knee that gets more tense after exercise. Felt as swelling or tightening.

CAUSE:
Fluid squeezes out backward in sac in knee. May leak internally, causing swelling in calf, ankle.

TREATMENT:
Self: Rest. Ignore if possible.
Medical: Do nothing. Leave alone. If necessary, aspirate and cortisone – treat any other cause of knee swelling. Surgery.

TRAINING:
Continue as usual.

BICEPS BURSA

Yes, one of the hamstring muscles is also called the biceps!

DIAGNOSIS:
Bony point on outside of knee is tender just under tendon or on tendon itself.

CAUSE:
Common in fast leg-action sports with fast high heel lift (i.e. sprinting).

TREATMENT:

Self: RICE.

Medical: Rest. Laser, ultrasound. Frictional massage. Cortisone injection. Check hamstring isokinetics.

TRAINING:

Continue as usual. Avoid repetition sprint sessions until better. Bend running (usually 200 m. 400 m.) on track may also make this flare up.

POPLITEUS STRAIN

DIAGNOSIS:

Pain from back of knee to outside of joint line.

CAUSE:

Twist of knee.

TREATMENT:

Self: Rest. There are too many nerves near to use ice.

Medical: Not common. Try rehabilitation. Take great care as major vessels nearby.

TRAINING:

Cycling, rowing, straight-line running until better.

LOWER LEG

Endurance training should be done on soft ground since constant running on hard roads and pavements jars the leg joints and bones and may lead to stress fractures. It is, of course, easier to run on firm ground, so try to save this sort of running for shorter, quality workouts. Try resting your bones and joints by doing endurance work on a bike or a rowing machine, etc.

The Achilles heel has a place in mythology with good reason: it causes most of the problems in this area of the body. Do not rush back to your sport before you have worked right through the specially designed Achilles ladder. Why play at 80 per cent fitness for the next year when proper treatment, allied to patience, can get you 100 per cent fit?

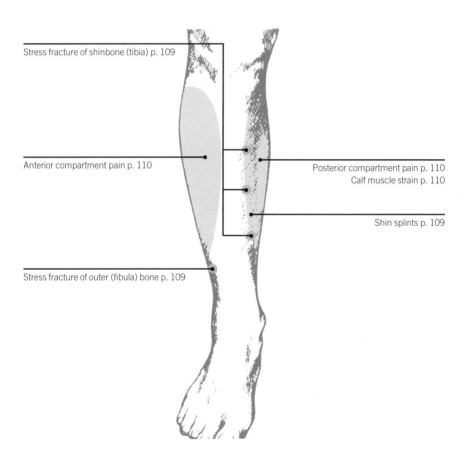

Stress fracture of shinbone (tibia) p. 109

Anterior compartment pain p. 110

Posterior compartment pain p. 110
Calf muscle strain p. 110

Shin splints p. 109

Stress fracture of outer (fibula) bone p. 109

LOWER LEG

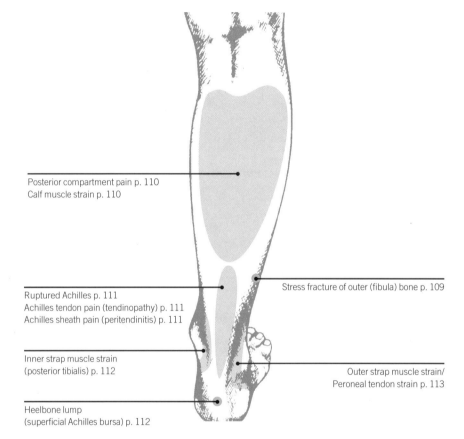

Posterior compartment pain p. 110
Calf muscle strain p. 110

Stress fracture of outer (fibula) bone p. 109

Ruptured Achilles p. 111
Achilles tendon pain (tendinopathy) p. 111
Achilles sheath pain (peritendinitis) p. 111

Inner strap muscle strain
(posterior tibialis) p. 112

Outer strap muscle strain/
Peroneal tendon strain p. 113

Heelbone lump
(superficial Achilles bursa) p. 112

STRESS FRACTURE OF SHINBONE (Tibia)

DIAGNOSIS:
Hurts on starting simple exercise such as running. Settles with rest. Painful to touch over small area (1 in./1-2 cm.). Painful to walk. Commonly found either one-third of the way down from knee or one third up from ankle, but also occurs midway between knee and ankle.

CAUSE:
Overuse, often increasing speed and/or distance too fast during training. A bounding style of running is more susceptible than shuffling, low-knee lift style. Also caused by knock-knees, turned-out feet, enthusiastic aerobics, jumping jacks with flat-footed landing.

TREATMENT:
Self: Rest from running for 5-6 weeks. *Medical:* Rest. Bone scan. Check posterior tibialis strength. Cortisone injection of periosteum. Orthotics.

TRAINING:
Avoid all running for 5-6 weeks. Maintain other fitness by swimming, rowing, bike routines. After 5 weeks, begin Hamstring ladder. Check that shoes are well padded, then avoid running on hard surfaces. Try a shorter stride pattern and ensure correct foot placement as you run.
See: Track and Field Athletics, Skating (Chapter 5).

STRESS FRACTURE OF OUTER (Fibula) BONE

DIAGNOSIS:
When running or walking, pain occurs approximately one hand's breadth above outside anklebone. Hurts to press.

CAUSE:
Running with weight on outside of foot, common to bowlegs, and landing pigeon-toed on ball of foot.

TREATMENT:
Self and Medical: As for Stress fracture of shinbone, above. May have tibio varus from anteverted hip, so hip exercises may help.

TRAINING:
As for Stress fracture of shinbone, but try to correct pigeon-toed gait.

SHIN SPLINTS

DIAGNOSIS:
Pain along inner or outer edge of shinbone. Worse after exercise. Area 1-3 in. (2-7 cm.) tender to pressure.

CAUSE:
Overuse strain, producing tearing and thickening of muscles at join along shinbone. May be accompanied by stress fracture.

TREATMENT:
Self: RICE.
Medical: Rest. Bone scan. Orthotics. Strengthen posterior tibialis. If no stress fracture, laser, ultrasound. Surgery.

TRAINING:
Achilles ladders. Heels. Build up mileage slowly. Upper body work as usual.

POSTERIOR COMPARTMENT PAIN

DIAGNOSIS:
Calf muscle painful during or after exercise, long exertion.

CAUSE:
Overuse of calf muscle. Leg muscle cannot expand in its tight sheath, reduces blood supply to muscle.

TREATMENT:
Self: RICE, especially ice and elevation. Painkillers.
Medical: RICE. Laser, ultrasound. Pressure studies. Surgery to release sheath, both deep and superficial compartment.

TRAINING:
Continue as usual, up to the edge of the pain barrier.

ANTERIOR COMPARTMENT PAIN

DIAGNOSIS:
Pain in muscles on front and outside of shin after exercise. Tender to press.

CAUSE:
Overuse of muscles that lift forefoot and toes off ground. Muscle cannot expand in its tight sheath.

TREATMENT:
Self: RICE, especially ice and elevation. Painkillers.
Medical: RICE. Laser, ultrasound. Pressure studies. Surgery to release sheath.

TRAINING:
Continue as usual, but avoid repeat work in hills, rough ground, long step-up sessions, sit-up holding with toes and feet.

See: Nerve irritation (p. 105). Skiing, Track and Field Athletics. (Chapter 5).

CALF MUSCLE STRAIN

DIAGNOSIS:
May feel like sudden kick or blow on calf. Hurts in calf when rising on tiptoe. Tender to press. May bruise.

CAUSE:
Overload tears calf muscle.

TREATMENT:
Self: RICE, especially compression, heel raise, crutches. Takes about 1-5 weeks to heal.
Medical: Laser, ultrasound. Massage, drain haematoma, cortisone.

TRAINING:
Upper body work as usual. Achilles ladders. Stretching exercises 1, 2, 9, 10, 11, 12 (especially 1, 2, 12).
See: Skiing (Chapter 5).

Achilles tendon

The tendon that runs from the calf to the heel is strong but does not have much blood supply, so while it does not tire, small tears and damage do not heal easily. With proper treatment, healing takes 4-16 weeks. The earlier an injury is treated, the better the result. Often the damage is a combination of Achilles tendinopathy (the tendon) and peritendinitis (the sheath). Most treatment helps the sheath; the tendon takes time and rehabilitation.

RUPTURED ACHILLES

DIAGNOSIS:
Sudden sharp pain may feel like kick or blow in leg. Cannot rise on tiptoe on that foot. Lie on bed face down, feet hanging over end; good foot has angle of 20-30° to vertical; bad foot hangs straight down at 90°. Squeeze calf with hand; good foot will move outward, bad foot will not move.

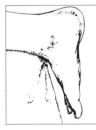 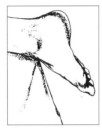

Ruptured achilles   Normal foot

CAUSE:
Tendon cannot take load and snaps.

TREATMENT:
Self: RICE. Insert heel raise in shoe. See doctor within 3-4 days.
Medical: Heel raise and plaster cast. Surgery.

TRAINING:
Supervised by doctor; Achilles ladders.

ACHILLES TENDON PAIN
(Tendinopathy)

DIAGNOSIS:
Pain in thick tendon of calf muscle. May develop lump if not allowed to heal properly. Hurts to rise on tiptoes; hurts to run; does not "run off".
See: Peritendinitis below, Ankle,

Jumper's/Dancer's heel.

CAUSE:
Minor tear or degeneration of Achilles tendon.

TREATMENT:
Self: RICE. Heel raise. Do not return to activities until training ladders completed. Hurrying back too soon will result in large scar and permanent pain.
Medical: Heel raise. Laser and ultrasound do not affect healing. MRI scan. Orthotics. Stretching. Rehabilitation. Surgery.
See: Achilles sheath pain.

TRAINING:
Achilles ladders. Stretching exercises 1, 2, 9, 10, 11, 12 (especially 1, 2, 12).

ACHILLES SHEATH PAIN
(Peritendinitis)

DIAGNOSIS:
Holding your foot in your hand, move the front (toe end) of it up and down; Achilles may grate, give pain over Achilles tendon. Stiff when sitting or first getting up in the morning; gets better the more you move around. Can "run it off", move around more comfortably when warmed up.

CAUSE:
Sometimes the high heel-tab, or so-called Achilles protector on sports shoes may press or jam into Achilles tendon, causing damage. This may occur even if you use athletic shoes as leisure wear. Often accompanies Achilles tendon pain (see above), producing thickening and roughening of Achilles tendon lining.

TREATMENT:
Self: RICE. Massage. NSAIDs gel. Cut off Achilles protector tab on shoes and tape down rough edge.
Medical: NSAIDs. Laser, ultrasound. Deep friction massage. Cortisone injection. Surgery.

TRAINING:
Achilles ladders. Stretching exercises 1, 2, 9 10, 11, 12 (especially 1, 2, 12).

HEELBONE LUMP
(Superficial Achilles bursa)

DIAGNOSIS:
Bony knob of heel is tender. Does not hurt to rise barefoot on tiptoe. May feel hot, look red and puffy.

CAUSE:
Shoe rubbing on skin of heel.

TREATMENT:
Self: RICE. NSAIDs gel. Stretch heel of shoe, cover with shiny plaster and soap outside of the plaster to allow shoe to slip. Try bigger shoe with two pairs of socks. "Second skin" type of plastic aid.
Medical: Laser, ultrasound. Cortisone injection. Orthotics. Surgery.

TRAINING:
Continue as usual. If sore to run, train with patter, bike routines with no shoes; swimming routine.

INNER STRAP MUSCLE STRAIN
(Posterior tibialis)

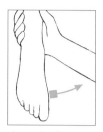

DIAGNOSIS:
Pain behind and beneath inner anklebone. May also extend down side of foot and underneath arch. Block inward movement of foot as shown in diagram; pain confirmed. May just be weak, with no pain.

CAUSE:
The muscle of the foot that balances you is strained when trying to counteract pronating feet. Rolling over on the inside of foot may strain this tendon and its sheath, especially in long-distance running, or incorrect pliés in ballet.

TREATMENT:
Self: Massage. Practise picking up a pencil with your toes to help raise the arch of your foot. Standing up, concentrate on pulling knees backward and outward using muscles only; keep your weight on the outside of foot, raising arch. Wear good shoes with strong heel cup and arch support; use a stirrup strap, as in the diagram, or a support ankle brace.
See: Ankle – Flat foot pain, Sprained ankle.
Medical: Laser, ultrasound. Cross-frictional massage. Cortisone injection. Orthotics. MR scan. Surgery.

TRAINING:
Rest from running. Bike, swimming, rowing routines. Build up running via Achilles top ladder.

OUTER STRAP MUSCLE STRAIN/PERONEAL TENDON STRAIN

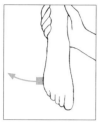

DIAGNOSIS:
Pain behind and under outer anklebone. May extend down outside of foot and underneath. Block outward movement of foot as shown; pain confirmed. May just be weak, with no pain.

CAUSE:
A strain on the balancing muscles of foot, often following twisted ankle; strain on muscles trying to counteract a pigeon-toed running gait or where weight is heavily on outside of foot. Tendon may slip over outside anklebone, causing "flicking" and pain.

TREATMENT:
Self: RICE. Massage tender areas. NSAIDs. Use stirrup strap (see diagram) but on outside of foot. Try cutting insole lengthwise and putting outer half in shoe to raise outer edge of foot.
Medical: Check for subluxing peroneal tendon, unstable ankle. Stress x-ray, brace. Laser, ultrasound. Cross frictional massage. Cortisone injection. Surgery. Orthotics.

TRAINING:
Avoid running until better. Swimming, bike, rowing routines. Build through Achilles top ladder.
See: Squash (Chapter 5), Home and Workplace (p. 156).

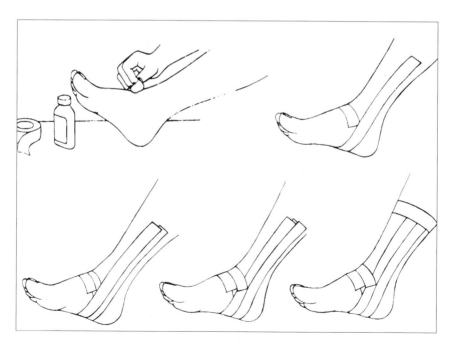

ANKLE

The stresses and strains of balancing, checking, turning and running on rough ground are all focused on this area, which is probably second only to the knee in vulnerability to injuries. Until recovery is complete, strapping to support the ligaments is helpful, as are orthotics, which can correct an unstable foot position and help with balance. Lace-up ankle braces are better than taping (and not as painful to remove), are re-usable and cheaper. Stronger braces support mildly unstable ankles.

WARNING

A difficult area to make accurate diagnosis, so consult doctor if any doubts. Also check diagnostic tests for Lower Leg (pp 109-110).

OUTSIDE

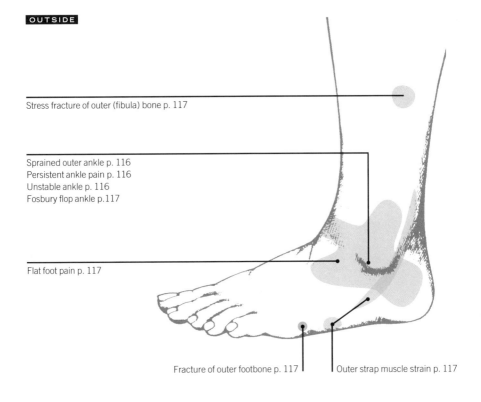

Stress fracture of outer (fibula) bone p. 117

Sprained outer ankle p. 116
Persistent ankle pain p. 116
Unstable ankle p. 116
Fosbury flop ankle p.117

Flat foot pain p. 117

Fracture of outer footbone p. 117   Outer strap muscle strain p. 117

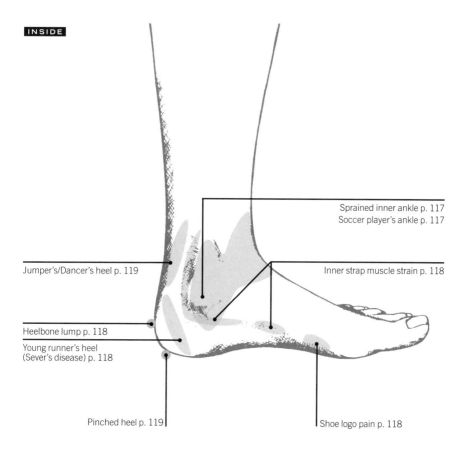

Sprained inner ankle p. 117
Soccer player's ankle p. 117

Jumper's/Dancer's heel p. 119

Inner strap muscle strain p. 118

Heelbone lump p. 118

Young runner's heel
(Sever's disease) p. 118

Pinched heel p. 119

Shoe logo pain p. 118

SPRAINED OUTER ANKLE

DIAGNOSIS:
Some or all of the following apply:
• Painful at rest.
• First few paces excruciating, then eases up while walking, but severe pain again on stopping.
• Red, swollen, bruising on side of foot, feels warm.

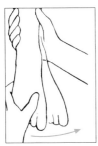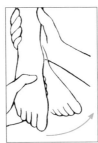

• Hurts when heelbone is moved inward or big toe pointed downward and inward (see diagrams).
• Hurts to touch.

CAUSE:
Turning ankle over onto outside of foot.

TREATMENT:
Self: RICE, especially compression and elevation. NSAIDs if severe. Avoid weight on ankle, use crutches for 48 hours. Support with strapping or ankle brace. Keep this on at night. Use cardboard box as cage to lift bedclothes off ankle. When start walking, maintain strapping; take smaller steps and try to walk heel/toe with foot pointing straight ahead; later, balance on leg while doing daily chores such as brushing teeth, telephoning, etc. Exercises as for Outer strap muscle strain (see under Lower Leg). Practise balance on wobble board (round platform attached to sphere).

Medical: RICE. Laser, ultrasound. Wobble board. Cross-frictional massage. Peroneal isometrics. Calcano cuboid may be involved. Treat as for above. May need manipulation and cortisone.

TRAINING:
Continue upper body work. Bike, rowing routines as soon as able. Wobble board. Knee ladder with ankle support. Maintain support for 6 weeks after resuming competition.
See: Basketball (Chapter 5).

PERSISTENT ANKLE PAIN

DIAGNOSIS:
Stiff, painful ankle movements persisting 4-6 weeks after sprained ankle. See diagnosis diagrams for sprained ankle.

CAUSE:
Ligaments heal but mobility of joint not fully restored. Scar tissue stiffens joint.

TREATMENT:
Self: Seek medical advice.
Medical: See Jumper's/Dancer's ankle. If stiff rather than unstable, manipulation, cortisone injection. If not stiff or unstable, check for loose bodies and particularly talar osteochondral lesion, then treat as for Sprained outer ankle.

TRAINING:
Continue as usual.

UNSTABLE ANKLE

DIAGNOSIS:
Only by doctor.

CAUSE:
Wrenched ankle.

TREATMENT:
Self: Support or brace.
Medical: Brace. Stress x-ray. Surgery.
TRAINING:
Under medical supervision, maintain quads; rowing, bike routines; then, patter routine, Achilles and Knee ladders.

FOSBURY FLOP ANKLE

See: Track and Field Athletics (Chapter 5).

OUTER STRAP MUSCLE STRAIN

See: Lower Leg.

FRACTURE OF OUTER FOOTBONE

DIAGNOSIS:
Only by doctor.
TREATMENT:
Medical: Beware Jones fracture, can suffer nonunion.

STRESS FRACTURE OF OUTER (Fibula) BONES

See: Lower Leg.

FLAT FOOT PAIN

DIAGNOSIS:
Pain over front of outside anklebone when pressed and also when foot lifted up and outward.
CAUSE:
Flat foot rolls inward, causing strain on inner strap muscle and joints. Running forces outside foot up into outer anklebone.

TREATMENT:
Self: When buying trainers, ask for antipronation shoes. Arch support, often with wedge under inside of heel and big toe joint. Good shoes strengthened with heel cup and inner support. Try stirrup strap (see diagram p. 113) starting on outside of foot, under, then up and over inside of ankle, correcting rolled-over arch. Practise picking up pencil in toes; standing up, tighten buttocks, draw knees back and outward, using muscles only. Practise regularly every day.
Medical: Arch support. Faradism to feet muscles. Posterior tibialis rehabilitation. Orthotics.
TRAINING:
Continue as usual, corrective mechanism in place.

SPRAINED INNER ANKLE

DIAGNOSIS:
Pain on and below inner anklebone. May have swelling and bruising that will discolour foot. Pain on forcing foot upward and outward (see diagrams).

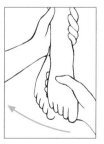 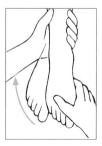

CAUSE:
Turning ankle over onto inside of foot. Not as common as outer ankle sprain. Check with doctor as fracture or unstable

rupture may occur.

TREATMENT:
Self: See: Sprained outer ankle.
Medical: See: Sprained outer ankle. X-ray. Chronic deltoid ligament, often needs cortisone injection.

TRAINING:
See: Sprained outer ankle.
See: Basketball, Handball, Netball, Volleyball (Chapter 5).

HEELBONE LUMP/PUMP BUMP

See: Lower Leg. Heelbone lump (p. 112).
Medical: Haglund syndrome.

SOCCER PLAYER'S ANKLE

DIAGNOSIS:
Thickened ankle area that may hurt to touch. May hurt to move or may be pain free. Often no trouble during game, stiff and aching afterwards.

CAUSE:
Repeated kicks, and sprain of ankle ligaments, from side foot tackle or blocked kick. X-rays reveal small fragments of bone and calcium.

TREATMENT:
Self: RICE. NSAIDs. Shin pads with ankle flaps, or felt/foam ankle padding under socks. May require brace.
Medical: RICE. NSAIDs. Manipulation and cortisone. Surgery.

TRAINING:
Continue as usual.
See: Basketball, Handball, Soccer (Chapter 5).

SHOE LOGO PAIN

DIAGNOSIS:
Sore area of skin; may even be rubbed raw. Usually hurts on inside of foot.

CAUSE:
Shoe manufacturer's logo or decorations are usually made of plastic and therefore do not expand with leather of shoe. This can cause pressure on foot near logo's attachment to sole.

TREATMENT:
Self: Slit across logo near attachment to sole of shoe.

INNER STRAP MUSCLE STRAIN

See under: Lower Leg.

YOUNG RUNNER'S HEEL
(Sever's disease)

DIAGNOSIS:
This is not a disease, but is peculiar to growing youngsters who train or participate too enthusiastically. Hurts as foot strikes ground, sometimes on take-off for jumping.

CAUSE:
Overuse damages "growing points" of heelbone.

TREATMENT:
Self: NSAIDs. Rest.
Medical: Rest. No long-term harm. Youngster can continue exercise as long as not limping.
See: How much training (p. 129). If pain occurs on take-off, then more rest required than for an impact pain. Interferential may help, as may air soles in shoes.

Save running for matches. In training, use swimming, biking, rowing routines. Build gently into patter routine if no pain, then use Achilles top ladder. Maintain quads and upper body strength throughout.

JUMPER'S/DANCER'S HEEL

DIAGNOSIS:
Pain on pressure between Achilles tendon and back of anklebones. Hurts on full pointes (ballet) or tiptoe. Hurts on take-off but not landing. Pain confirmed by forcibly jamming heel against back of shinbone, by snapping foot downward into pointes.

CAUSES:
• Repeatedly rising on tiptoe (dancer's pointes).
• Explosive jumping, such as basketball, high jump, triple jump.
• Foot blocked as ball is kicked with toes pointing downward.
• Stamping heel down when finishing movement.
• In the first four causes, a pad of fat is compressed between heelbone and shinbone. Sometimes, however, a bone (os trigonum) is present, like a nut between nutcrackers.
• May accompany severe ankle sprain when bruising comes on inside and outside of ankle because ligaments at back of ankle joint damaged as well as normal sprained ankle.

TREATMENT:
Self: Rest. NSAIDs. Avoid movements that point the toes to the floor.

Medical: NSAIDs. X-ray to exclude os trigonum and unstable ankle joint. Laser, ultrasound. Interferential. Cortisone injection. Surgical removal of os trigonum bone.

TRAINING:
Avoid pointes, jumping (high, long and triple jump) and bounding routines if sore. Exercise probably safe but pain will recur. Maintain heel exercises within pain free range. Use Achilles ladder. See: Soccer, Basketball (Chapter 5).

PINCHED HEEL

DIAGNOSIS:
Painful skin and soft tissue under back of heel.

CAUSE:
Bruising of skin and pad of fat under heelbone.

TREATMENT:
Self: Insert firmer heel cup to shoe and large absorbent heel, or use absorbent rubber heel pads.
Medical: Rest.

TRAINING:
Continue as usual if no pain.

FOOT AND TOES

Athlete's foot and blisters may be the most familiar foot problems, but more serious and often ignored are the overuse injuries caused by stress on the many small bones that have to take the whole weight of the body. Good shoes for daily wear, as well as sports and leisure, are vital. Orthotics may help correct some problems but must always be fitted by an expert.

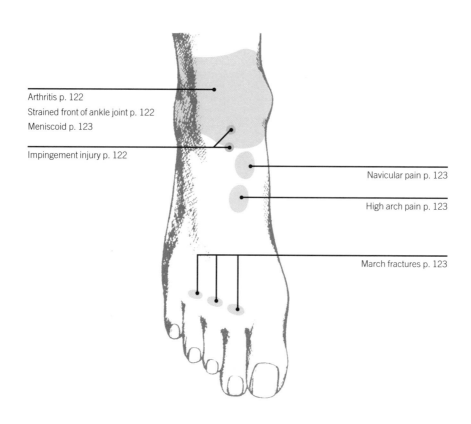

Arthritis p. 122
Strained front of ankle joint p. 122
Meniscoid p. 123

Impingement injury p. 122

Navicular pain p. 123

High arch pain p. 123

March fractures p. 123

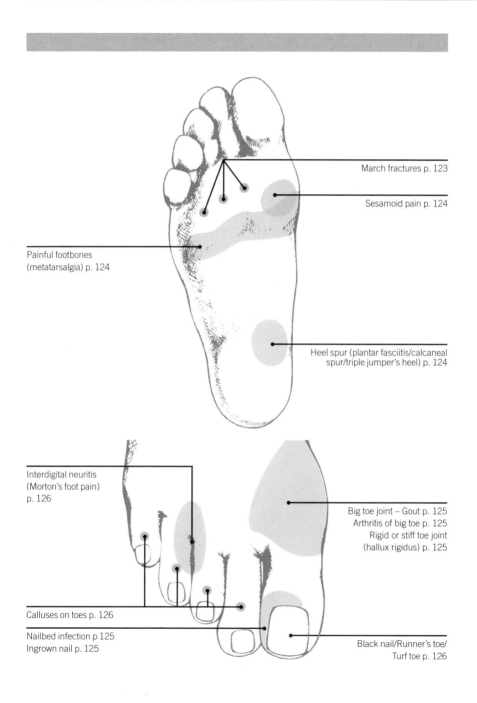

March fractures p. 123

Sesamoid pain p. 124

Painful footbones
(metatarsalgia) p. 124

Heel spur (plantar fasciitis/calcaneal
spur/triple jumper's heel) p. 124

Interdigital neuritis
(Morton's foot pain)
p. 126

Big toe joint – Gout p. 125
Arthritis of big toe p. 125
Rigid or stiff toe joint
(hallux rigidus) p. 125

Calluses on toes p. 126

Nailbed infection p 125
Ingrown nail p. 125

Black nail/Runner's toe/
Turf toe p. 126

ARTHRITIS

DIAGNOSIS:
May hurt at rest. Hurts to walk or run. All movements limited and painful at end of range. May cause swelling.

CAUSE:
As cartilage wears down, bones roughen from grating together.

TREATMENT:
Self: Rest. NSAIDs.
Medical: NSAIDs. Shortwave diathermy. Cortisone injection. X-ray or CT scan to exclude osteochondritis or loose body. Surgery.

TRAINING:
Total rest makes the condition worse, just as lots of high-impact exercise makes worse. Best to carry on with low-impact exercise such as swimming, cycling, rowing. May signal end of really active sports/games.

STRAINED FRONT OF ANKLE JOINT

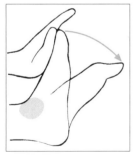

DIAGNOSIS:
Most movements of ankle are painless apart from forcing foot downward. See: Meniscoid.

CAUSE:
Strain of ligaments by sudden major, or repeated minor blows to foot. Forcing foot downward, for example, by kicking a ball or having a kick blocked.

TREATMENT:
Self: Rest. NSAIDs. Double stirrup strapping (see p. 113).
Medical: Prolonged rest. Shortwave diathermy. Laser, ultrasound. Cross-frictional massage. Cortisone injection. Strapping.

TRAINING:
Continue as usual. Avoid kicking. See: Soccer (Chapter 5).

IMPINGEMENT INJURY

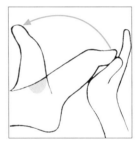

DIAGNOSIS:
Tender to touch near top part of foot. Hurts when foot forced up as far as possible.

CAUSE:
Upper foot bones bang or impinge against shinbone, causing pain and sometimes producing spurs of bone which can fracture.

TREATMENT:
Self: Rest.
Medical: Rest. Cortisone injection. Surgery.

TRAINING:
Continue as usual. See: Badminton, Gymnastics (Chapter 5).

MENISCOID

DIAGNOSIS:
See: Strained front of ankle joint and Impingement injury.

CAUSE:
Blood vessels and joint lining become swollen and thickened from either of above causes.

TREATMENT:
Self: NSAIDs.
Medical: Cortisone injection. Surgery.

TRAINING:
As normal; avoid movement that makes worse.

NAVICULAR PAIN

DIAGNOSIS:
May hurt to walk, trot, run, but certainly to sprint. Foot movements are pain free but pressure over upper inner foot bone hurts.

CAUSE:
Stress fracture, usually in sprints, long or triple jump events.

TREATMENT:
Self: Rest.
Medical: Rest. Crutches. Bone or CT scan. Plaster cast. May be slow to heal, prone to non-union. Surgery.

TRAINING:
No running. Do swimming, bike, rowing routines. Try Achilles top ladder when healed.

HIGH ARCH PAIN

DIAGNOSIS:
Pain and sometimes swelling on highest part of foot. Hurts to touch, but all foot movements pain free. Worse in shoes.

CAUSE:
Pressure because shape of shoe not cut with enough room for high arch.

TREATMENT:
Self: Apply ice to affected part. Loosen laces. Get new pair of shoes or stretch old ones. Check that shoe inserts or orthotics are not taking up too much space.
Medical: As above.

TRAINING:
Continue as usual.

MARCH FRACTURES

DIAGNOSIS:
Pain in central bones of forefoot when walking, marching (origin of name), trotting, running. Hurts to press relevant bone both from top and from sole of foot.

CAUSE:
Stress fracture of metatarsals.

TREATMENT:
Self: Rest. Use firm shoes for everyday wear which act like a splint around foot bones; get shoes with really absorbent soles and inners.
Medical: Rest. X-ray. Bone scan.

TRAINING:
Avoid running, even walking. Do swimming, bike, rowing routines later. Try Achilles top ladder.

HEEL SPUR
(Plantar fasciitis/Calcaneal spur/Triple jumper's heel)

DIAGNOSIS:
Hurts under heel to walk or run. Painful to pressure. Half rising on ball of foot may hurt heel.

CAUSE:
Strain of spring ligament of a heel bone caused either by banging of heel or jumping at half-stretch as in badminton smash. Spur of bone may be seen on x-ray but may not be cause of the problem.

TREATMENT:
Self: Rest. Insert shock-absorbent heel pads at least ¼ in. (½ cm.) thick when compressed. Firm heel cup. NSAIDs. Also try arch support.
Medical: Rest. Heel pads. Corrective orthotic. Cortisone injection. Stretch and work spring ligament. NSAIDs, especially if gout or spondylarthropathy. Check medial calcaneal nerve.

TRAINING:
Upper body work as usual. Swimming, rowing, bike, patter routines. Run when pain free.
See: Badminton, Track and Field Athletics (Chapter 5).

PAINFUL FOOTBONES (Metatarsalgia)

DIAGNOSIS:
Painful bones on ball of foot when running or walking. Hurts to press and may have prominent callous on skin. See also March fracture.

CAUSE:
Banging foot down on ground bruises the more prominent bones. More common in feet with high arches, claw toes and in older people. Foot imbalance may cause pain under inside or outside of foot.

TREATMENT:
Self: Cut pad of felt and place just behind forefoot bones. The pad lifts up the forefoot and flattens claw toes, larger shoes may be needed as result.
Medical: Metatarsal pad. Orthotics. Check for osteochondritis in children. Surgery.

TRAINING:
Continue as usual, unless painful.

SESAMOID PAIN

DIAGNOSIS:
Pain on ball of foot under big toe. Hurts to run or walk. Hurts to touch. Also hurts to resist gripping movement of big toe.

CAUSE:
Banging or hard landing on small bone in tendon to big toe joint. This produces bruising or even fracture, especially in fast acceleration sports or with sports with fast changes of direction such as tennis, squash, badminton.

TREATMENT:
Self: Rest. NSAIDs.
Medical: NSAIDs. Laser, ultrasound. Cortisone injection. Plaster cast. Can be fracture.

TRAINING:
Continue as usual unless painful.

Toes

See: Tennis (Chapter 5).

BIG TOE JOINT/GOUT

DIAGNOSIS:
Hot, swollen joint. Painful at rest and to move in any direction.

NOTE
This can occur in other joints in body.

CAUSE:
Upset in body chemistry, perhaps from eating too much meat. Unlikely in pre-menopausal women.

TREATMENT:
Self: Rest. NSAIDs.
Medical: NSAIDs, allopurinol. Note probenecid is banned for sports.

TRAINING:
Rest.

ARTHRITIS OF BIG TOE

DIAGNOSIS:
May be painful at rest. Walking and running may hurt. Hurts at end of range of all movements.

CAUSE:
As cartilage wears down, bones roughen from grating together.

TREATMENT:
Self: Rest. NSAIDs. Warm bath. Run/walk with foot turned slightly outward with a shorter stride to avoid rising up and over big toe; runners may have to alter to more shuffling gait.
Medical: NSAIDs. Orthotics. Interferential. Shortwave diathermy. Cortisone injection. Surgery.

TRAINING:
Continue as usual.

RIGID OR STIFF TOE JOINT (Hallux rigidus)

DIAGNOSIS:
Big toe has little or no movement either up or down. May or may not be painful.

CAUSE:
Big toe goes completely stiff.

TREATMENT:
Self: As for Arthritis.
Medical: As for Arthritis, Use metatarsal bar.

TRAINING:
Continue as usual.
See: Tennis (Chapter 5).

NAILBED INFECTION

DIAGNOSIS:
Red, painful, swollen, even with white or yellow area surrounding base and on side of nail.

CAUSE:
Infection in skin.

TREATMENT:
Self: Seek medical advice. Firm strapping may ease pain. Release pus by sterilizing needle in flame until red hot, cooling, then opening skin only through yellow or white area.
Medical: Drain pus. Antibiotics. Surgery.

TRAINING:
Rest until cured.

INGROWN NAIL

DIAGNOSIS:
Pain, redness and discharge down side

of nail and also near cut edge.

CAUSE:

Nail edge damages skin, causing infection.

TREATMENT:

Self: Cut nails square with very slight rounding; over-rounded nail may leave spear that grows into skin. Pack cotton wool between nail and skin fold. Try to cut off spear of nail. Seek medical advice.
Medical: Antibiotics. Packing of nail. Surgery.

TRAINING:

Continue as usual.

BLACK NAIL/RUNNER'S TOE/ TURF TOE

DIAGNOSIS:

Nail starts to turn black near base. May be painful. If this occurs rapidly, may be very painful and throbbing. Joint may also be swollen and painful; hurts in all movements and may have bone damage.

CAUSE:

• Shoe too short or does not hold width of foot firmly so that foot slides forward and jams against end of shoe, especially on dry artificial turf.
• Blow to toe may immediately bruise, causing blood under pressure beneath nail, which is very painful. Nail later dies and grows out to drop off. Black area grows away from nailbed to end of nail.

TREATMENT:

Self: RICE. NSAIDs. Heat pin, hold in tweezers, burn hole in nail. This doesn't hurt, but releases spurt of blood; pain subsides. Try padding tongue of shoe with felt to stop forward slip of foot. Try

new shoes.
Medical: NSAIDs. Shortwave diathermy. Drain blood through hole in nail as above. Antibiotics.

TRAINING:

Continue as usual.
See: Hockey (field), Squash (Chapter 5).

CALLUSES ON TOES

DIAGNOSIS:

Thickened pads on top of toe joints. See diagram of toes. Painful foot bones.

CAUSE:

Either claw toes or shoes too short.

TREATMENT:

Self: Try metatarsal pad. Longer pair of shoes.
See: Painful foot bones.
Medical: Metatarsal pad. Surgery.

TRAINING:

Continue as usual.

INTERDIGITAL NEURITIS (Morton's foot pain)

DIAGNOSIS:

Burning pain down side of adjacent toes, usually 2nd and 3rd or 3rd and 4th toes. Worse when squeezing width of foot.

CAUSE:

Trapped nerve.

TREATMENT:

Self: Arch support and pad as for Painful foot bones Metatarsalgia. Wider shoes.
Medical: Cortisone injection. Orthotics. Check March fracture. Possible neuroma. Surgery.

TRAINING:

Continue as usual.

4

How to Recover From an Injury

DR. MALCOLM READ'S TRAINING LADDERS FOR REHABILITATION

Far too many recreational athletes, as well as professionals, rush back into action too soon, impatient after even the shortest lay-off. The result is often a recurrence of the problem or, as the athlete tries to favour the old injury, a new and different one.

The secret of a successful comeback is to put the injured area through a graduated series of exercises, each one a little more demanding than the last. This is how and why the following training ladders were devised. They have been used successfully by everyone from ballroom dancers to ballet dancers, from typists to taxi drivers, from weekend golfers to world and Olympic champions. The principles are always the same.

Starting on the bottom step of the ladder, the injured person works his or her way through these prescribed exercises. It is important to realize that all movement is a skill; in a simple form of exercise such as running there is a rhythm and balance between each leg. Loss of rhythm during rehabilitation may indicate, that in order to reach the training target, the body is using other muscles to protect the injured one. It is important to carry out the exercises correctly and to stop at the first sign of pain. If pain occurs, you may be damaging the injury further. If the pain or ache goes away after 20 seconds, the exercises may be continued. If the ache or pain persists, STOP – WAIT 24 hours – BEGIN AGAIN FROM THE FIRST STEP.

If there is a loss of rhythm, stay at the same level or drop back one step on the ladder to regain rhythm. Do not push on to the next level, even if there is no pain.

The new session should start from the bottom but, when reaching a higher level, you may cut down on the number of repetitions.

No two injuries are alike, so the rate of healing will vary from person to person. By using these training ladders, any athlete can assess when he or she has done too much. To find out which ladder plan is right for you, first diagnose your injury using the Top-to-Toe Guide in Chapter 3. Correct treatment and training is given there, referring you to the appropriate ladder plan if necessary. Legs receive the most injuries, so there are several different ladders dealing with specific leg injuries. Some have two stages, a lower, and an upper ladder. The lower ladder is designed to keep you fit in the early stages of recovery, while the upper concentrates on rebuilding the strength and technique required by the legs. However, the lower should still be used after you have graduated to the upper ladder. Everyone from soccer players to netball players and hockey players to sprinters can use these.

Other sports, like tennis, badminton, squash and baseball, require special rehabilitation ladders for the arms. These are also included. The General muscle ladder spells out the principles that apply to any injury, setting out a step-by-step return to full match fitness.

How much training to do when injured

- Intensity should just reach the point of pain. Stop, allow pain to settle, then continue. If the pain lasts 20-30 seconds, stop. Train again next day.
- If injury doesn't hurt at time but hurts later, use NSAIDs.

(a) If pain settled by following morning, then training is within injury tolerance.

(b) If pain is worse the following morning, but settles by midday, you are training at the maximum, so reduce the load.

(c) If the pain is worse for the following 24-48 hours, then you have been training well over the maximum recommended. Rest until settled. Start again, with a considerable reduction in your load.

- If you are making good progress, do not increase speed and distance or weight and number of repetitions at same time. Increase distance first, later speed; number of repetitions first, then weight.

NOTE

Always stretch properly before exercises.

Cross-training routines

Training using sports different to your own helps to protect all injuries but, at the same time, keeps you fit. The different routines referred to in the ladder plans are explained below.

PATTER ROUTINE

This simple exercise is effective in raising pulse rate, building fitness without straining knees or hips. It also takes up very little time: quality not quantity is vital in fitness training.

The secret is in not lifting the feet far off the ground. What we call a slow patter is more like fast jogging on the spot with knees kept low. Feet must be lifted only 1-2 in. (2.5-5 cm.) off the floor. A fast patter has the same low knee and foot lift, but you must patter as fast as you can. It is testing yet simple.

Routine for unfit athlete (3 minutes)

1 min.	slow patter
5 sec.	fast patter
50 sec.	slow patter
5 sec.	fast patter
50 sec.	slow patter
10 sec.	fast patter

Rest for 3 minutes while doing stretching exercises. Repeat above routine at least twice, preferably four times.

Routine for fairly fit athlete (5 minutes)

50 sec.	slow patter
10 sec.	fast patter
40 sec.	slow patter
20 sec.	fast patter
50 sec.	slow patter
10 sec.	fast patter
30 sec.	slow patter
10 sec.	fast patter
50 sec.	slow patter
30 sec.	fast patter

Rest for 3 minutes while doing stretching exercises. Repeat above routine at least once, preferably three times.

Routine for fit athlete (13 minutes)

Do routine for unfit athlete once, followed immediately by routine for fairly fit athlete twice.

SKIPPING ROUTINE

If you are good at skipping, try to use the same timing as the above patter routines. This gives the calf muscles a particularly good workout.

SWIMMING ROUTINE

Swimming is an excellent way to keep the muscles toned up, especially when you cannot run through injury. The water supports the body's weight but does not offer great resistance. Although less muscle power is required, the pulse rate is still raised by swimming. Try to run in water, using a flotation jacket for stability. Don't just run with a high knee; try to take large strides, really pulling with the hamstrings.

Routine for poor swimmer/non-swimmer

Jump in, swim or flounder across the width of the pool, climb out using good leg, stand up. Now turn around and repeat the routine for 3-5 minutes. Rest for 3 minutes while doing stretching exercises. Repeat above routine at least twice, preferably four times.

Routine for good swimmer

As above but swim one length of the pool each time.

ROWING ROUTINE

You need a rowing machine or ergometric machine (not a real rowing boat) for this. It gives a thorough workout for legs, arms and abdominal muscles and builds stamina. Untrained rowers will find this much harder work than expected! Make sure you:

- Press equally hard with both legs. Try to get both knees to travel at same rate, especially when locking them straight.
- Lie back at end of stroke to exercise stomach muscles.
- Vary hand grip (either over top or underneath) if muscles ache.
- Each machine has a different pull, so adjust your own routines accordingly.
- If you have knee problems, do not throw knee out to the side. Try to keep knees in line with first and second toes as you move backward and forward. Drawing a mark over midline of kneecap will help you see if you waver around.

Routine for long-distance/Stamina events

Work so that you can still carry on a conversation, even if you are panting a bit. At least 10 minutes, though more than 30 minutes preferable.

Routine for middle-distance events and running ball games

2 minutes long distance, 1 minute sprint so that you don't have enough breath to chat. Rest 3 minutes. Repeat as often as you like.

Routines for sprint events and martial arts

At least 30 strokes per minute for 1-2 minutes. Rest 5 minutes. Repeat as often as you like.

BIKING ROUTINE

This takes the pressure off leg joints and avoids jarring the back but still allows excellent workout for heart and lungs. It may be done on a stationary exercise bike in a gym or on an ordinary pedal bike out on the road.

• For stamina training: Use easy, low gears at a pace where you are able to talk with only a slight pant.

• For sprint training: Use harder, higher gears. You should be unable to talk.

• Knee problems: Do not throw knee inward or outward; keep knees vertical over first and second toes; do not drop inside this line during pedalling.

Routine for long-distance running

Your time on the bike should be equal to the time you would normally spend training on foot, but you should cover a much longer distance, preferably 2 to 2½ times longer than you would usually run.

Routine for middle-distance running and ball games (5 minutes)

4½ min.	stamina training
½ min.	sprint training

Rest for 3 minutes while doing stretching exercises. Repeat at least twice, preferably four times.

Routine for sprint events, strength events, volleyball, basketball, etc. (5 minutes)

2 min.	stamina training
15 sec.	sprint training
1¾ min.	stamina training
1 min.	sprint training

Rest for 4 minutes while doing stretching exercises. Repeat at least twice, preferably four times.

ISOMETRICS

Isometrics is a word commonly used in sport. Although it sounds modern and trendy, it is actually the type of exercise that Charles Atlas made popular half a century ago. In isometrics, muscles are tensed, rather than stretched, and strengthened without lifting weights. For example, you can sit at a heavy desk and try to lift it. This would build your biceps. Isometrics can be done anytime, anywhere: in an elevator or on a subway, on a beach or in the garden.

Dr. Read's Rule of 7

• Push/tense for 7 seconds
• Rest for 7 seconds
• Repeat 7 times
• Do this 3-5 times a day.

GENERAL MUSCLE LADDER

At levels 7-8 of the General muscle ladder, use closed chain work for legs rather than, or as well as, open chain work. Balance on one leg, lower body weight over bent knee (knee over foot), straighten knee.
Open chain work means sitting leg curls or presses.

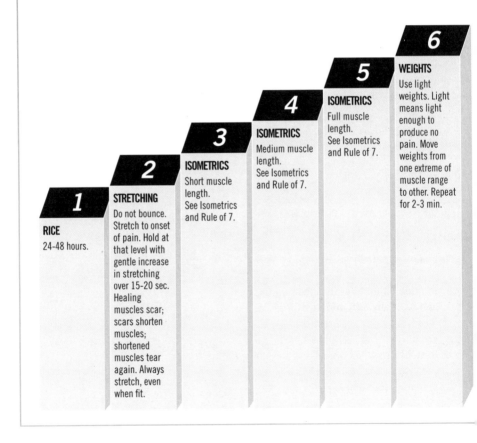

1

RICE
24-48 hours.

2

STRETCHING
Do not bounce. Stretch to onset of pain. Hold at that level with gentle increase in stretching over 15-20 sec. Healing muscles scar; scars shorten muscles; shortened muscles tear again. Always stretch, even when fit.

3

ISOMETRICS
Short muscle length. See Isometrics and Rule of 7.

4

ISOMETRICS
Medium muscle length. See Isometrics and Rule of 7.

5

ISOMETRICS
Full muscle length. See Isometrics and Rule of 7.

6

WEIGHTS
Use light weights. Light means light enough to produce no pain. Move weights from one extreme of muscle range to other. Repeat for 2-3 min.

7

INCREASE WEIGHTS

Increase load only to point that produces no pain.

8

TECHNICAL SKILL

Start technical skills slowly – e.g., running, swimming, throwing, hitting, etc. Do not lose rhythm and balance.

9

INCREASE FORCE

Practise techniques at half maximum effort. Do not lose rhythm.

10

MAXIMUM FORCE

Use maximum effort in practice. Do not lose rhythm. Do pleiometrics: hopping, bounding and depth jumps.

11

START PLAY

Begin in easy, low-grade match, easy opposition. Do pleiometrics: hopping, bounding and depth jumps.

12

FIT AGAIN!

Play at normal grade.

QUADS LADDER – STRENGTH

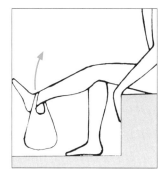

STEP 2

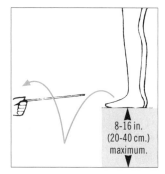

8-16 in.
(20-40 cm.)
maximum.

STEP 8

1

ISOMETRICS

Stand up, lock injured knee straight; tense thigh muscles. Rule of 7.

2

KNEE STRAIGHTENING

Support upper leg of injured knee on bench, in hands or on fit leg. Sit with bag containing 4½ lb. (2 kg.) hooked over ankle of injured leg. (Use bags of sugar.) Raise and straighten leg. Hold 10 sec. Repeat as needed.

3

SKIER'S EXERCISE

"Sit" with back against wall, thighs parallel to ground. Do not drop below horizontal. Hold 7 sec. Rest 7 sec. Repeat 7 times. Knees should remain over feet.

4

SLOW STEP-UPS

Step up and back onto a low bench or step, alternating feet.

5

LEG PRESS MACHINE

If available, use leg press machine in gym with light weights. Knee extension machines are not so good for cruciate injuries. Start closed chain balance knee bends. See: General muscle ladder or trainer.

6

SQUATS

If available, use weight-lifting squat technique. Use light weights, make sure knees never bend below 90°.

7

BIKE ROUTINE

Use high gear, low pedal rate. Continue until muscle aches. Rest 5-10 min. Repeat as fitness allows. Try seat at varying heights to make knee work straighter or more bent. Maintain strength; do not favour injured leg. Keep knee vertically above foot.

8

DEPTH JUMPS

Jump down from low step (6-8 in./15-20 cm.) then up over string or bar (e.g., high jump bar). Find highest you can jump. Drop this height by 2 in. (5 cm.), then repeat 10 times. Jump rhythmically down and over with no bounce in between. Start with both legs. Eventually improve to single-leg jumps. Over the weeks gradually raise height of step by placing, say, large book on it, but not more than 16 in. (40 cm.) high.

9

HOP, STEP, JUMP

Idea is to travel as far as you can. As this is measurable, you can have competitions with other recuperating athletes. Start with right toe on line, hop onto right foot, step onto left foot, jump from left foot, land on both feet or hop, hop, hop, etc. Mark how far you have gone. Repeat, starting from left foot. Do 5 times each foot.

10

WEIGHTS

Resume normal weight training to level before injury.

QUADS LADDER – HEART AND LUNGS

The Heart and Lungs ladder builds up your stamina. To rebuild muscle strength, use the Strength ladder. These two may be worked in parallel. However, competitors in power events should concentrate on strength, while speed and endurance competitors will find the Heart and Lungs ladder more appropriate. Competitors in most ball games (soccer, basketball, football, etc) will use both ladders.

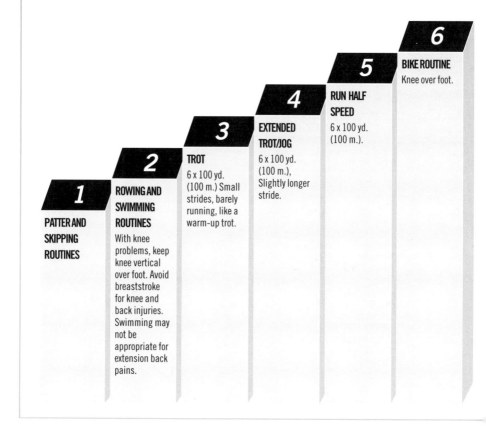

6
BIKE ROUTINE
Knee over foot.

5
RUN HALF SPEED
6 x 100 yd. (100 m.).

4
EXTENDED TROT/JOG
6 x 100 yd. (100 m.), Slightly longer stride.

3
TROT
6 x 100 yd. (100 m.) Small strides, barely running, like a warm-up trot.

2
ROWING AND SWIMMING ROUTINES
With knee problems, keep knee vertical over foot. Avoid breaststroke for knee and back injuries. Swimming may not be appropriate for extension back pains.

1
PATTER AND SKIPPING ROUTINES

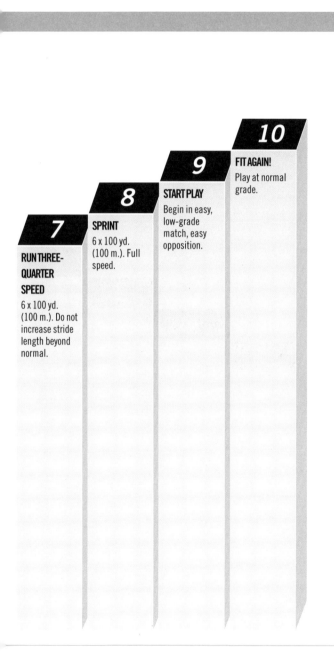

7

RUN THREE-QUARTER SPEED

6 x 100 yd. (100 m.). Do not increase stride length beyond normal.

8

SPRINT

6 x 100 yd. (100 m.). Full speed.

9

START PLAY

Begin in easy, low-grade match, easy opposition.

10

FIT AGAIN!

Play at normal grade.

KNEE LADDER

Knee should be supported (strapped or braced) through all of this ladder and for first 6 weeks of match play. When you can sprint 100 yd. (100 m.) without pain (i.e. at level 7 of Calf and Achilles or Hamstring top ladders), start here.

Kicking can start from level 1.
Using soccer ball:
1 6 ft. (2 m.) away from wall, side foot and instep
2 20 ft. (6 m.) from wall
3 With a partner, gradually move further apart

Using football:
4 Kicking from hand (caressing the ball)
5 Hard punt/kick
6 Hard kick from ground.

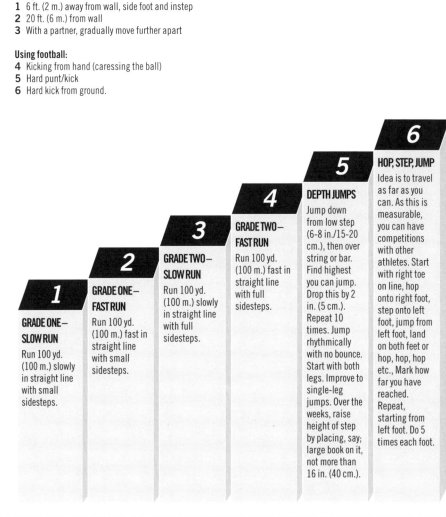

1

**GRADE ONE –
SLOW RUN**

Run 100 yd. (100 m.) slowly in straight line with small sidesteps.

2

**GRADE ONE –
FAST RUN**

Run 100 yd. (100 m.) fast in straight line with small sidesteps.

3

**GRADE TWO –
SLOW RUN**

Run 100 yd. (100 m.) slowly in straight line with full sidesteps.

4

**GRADE TWO –
FAST RUN**

Run 100 yd. (100 m.) fast in straight line with full sidesteps.

5

DEPTH JUMPS

Jump down from low step (6-8 in./15-20 cm.), then over string or bar. Find highest you can jump. Drop this by 2 in. (5 cm.). Repeat 10 times. Jump rhythmically with no bounce. Start with both legs. Improve to single-leg jumps. Over the weeks, raise height of step by placing, say, large book on it, not more than 16 in. (40 cm.).

6

HOP, STEP, JUMP

Idea is to travel as far as you can. As this is measurable, you can have competitions with other athletes. Start with right toe on line, hop onto right foot, step onto left foot, jump from left foot, land on both feet or hop, hop, hop etc., Mark how far you have reached. Repeat, starting from left foot. Do 5 times each foot.

9

FIT AGAIN!

Play at normal grade.

8

START PLAY

Begin in easy, low-grade match, easy opposition.

7

SHUTTLE RUN

10 x 20 yd. (20 m.) wind sprints. Sprint out and back in between markers 20 yd. (20 m.) apart.

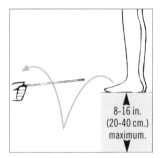

8-16 in. (20-40 cm.) maximum.

CALF AND ACHILLES BOTTOM LADDER

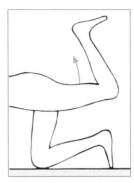

STEP 4

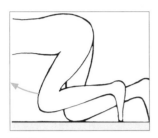

STEP 6

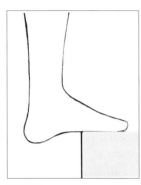

STEP 9

6

HEELS
Standing on ground with both feet together, raise your heels. Build up until you do 20. **Do not work** through pain. Do 20 standing on one leg. Progress to stairs. (See Hamstring bottom ladder.) After reaching 20 without pain, try standing on one leg. Start steps 7-8 on the ladder.

5

SWIMMING AND ROWING ROUTINES

4

BUTTOCK STRENGTH
On all fours on ground, bring knee up to chest, then swing leg back and up. Heel swings toward back of head! Repeat for 1-3 min. with both legs.

3

STRETCHING
Use stretching exercises 1, 2, 8, 9, 12 (Chapter 1). Remember to stretch until you feel pain. Hold for count of 15-20 sec. Breathe out. Repeat sequence 5 or 6 times a day. Do not bounce.

2

TOE POINTING
Sitting down with foot off ground, knee straight, point toe firmly downward, then upward to stretch Achilles tendon and calf muscle. Physiotherapy may now begin, also upper body exercises, sit-ups. Start steps 3 and 4.

1

RICE
24-48 hours. Place heel wedge or pad in everyday shoes. Cut rubber sponge if necessary. Women could wear high heels.

7

BIKE ROUTINE
During early
days of Achilles
injury, ball of
foot may be too
sore to use on
pedal. Use arch
until ball of foot
pain free. If
rowing and bike
machines
available in
gym, switch
from one to
other after rest
period – e.g.
bike 3 min., rest
3 min., row 3
min. (early in
injury may not
be able to come
forward too
far), rest 3
min., etc.

8

BIKE ROUTINE
Use ball of foot
(when pain
free).

9

HEELS
If strong
enough, start to
exercise one leg
at a time.

10

HOP
If you can hop
50 times on
injured leg and
feel no pain,
move to Top
ladder. This is a
test not a
training
session.

CALF AND ACHILLES TOP LADDER

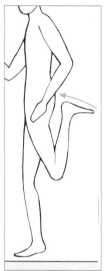

STEP 3

Start each training session from the bottom of the ladder. Early ladder steps may be cut from 6 to 3 repetitions. Continue using Calf and Achilles bottom ladder for fitness. Check that leg rhythm is always equal; do not gallop. One way to avoid favouring injured leg is to count out loud from 1 to 9 while running. This sets rhythm for legs to follow and allows concentration to move from one leg to the other. Counting 1, 2; 1, 2 tends to stress any limp. Do stretching exercises between each 100 yd. (100 m.). Check knee lift and heel pickup are same height. Stop if pain lasts more than 20-30 seconds, or if there is a loss of rhythm.

1 TROT
6 x 100 yd. (100 m.). Small stride barely running, like a warm-up trot.

2 EXTENDED TROT/JOG
6 x 100 yd. (100 m.) Slightly longer stride.

3 HIGH HEELS
6 x 100 yd. (100 m.). Trot with heels deliberately kicking buttocks on each stride. This works hamstring and also keeps you longer on balls of feet.

4 RUN HALF SPEED
6 x 100 yd. (100 m.).

5 HIGH KNEE TROT
6 x 100 yd. (100 m.). Keep stride length short, knees raised to horizontal or above. Non-sprinters can make do with half this distance.

6 RUN HALF SPEED
6 x 100 yd. (100 m.). Do not stretch to increase stride length beyond normal. Do not bound.

12

FIT AGAIN!

Play at normal grade.

11

START PLAY

Begin in easy, low-grade match, easy opposition.

10

SHUTTLE RUN

10 x 20 yd. (20 m.) wind sprints. Sprint out and back in between markers 20 yd. (20 m.) apart.

9

GRADE THREE SPRINT

6 x 100 yd. (100 m.). Fast accelerate 25 yd. (25 m.); sprint 50 yd. (50 m.); fast stop 25 yd. (25 m.).

8

GRADE TWO SPRINT

6 x 100 yd. (100 m.). Accelerate 25 yd. (25 m.); sprint 50 yd. (50 m.); fast stop 25 yd. (25 m.).

Note: Specialist runners should still use slow stop (step 7). Fast stop is only for stop-start sports, usually ball games.

7

GRADE ONE SPRINT

6 x 100 yd. (100 m.). Accelerate 25 yd. (25 m.); sprint 50 yd. (50 m.); slow down 25 yd. (25 m.).

HAMSTRING BOTTOM LADDER

If the knee is injured, particularly anterior cruciate and ligaments, it should be supported (strapped/braced) throughout all of this ladder work and for the first 6 weeks of match play.

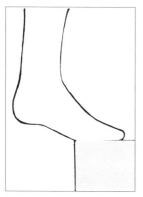

STEP 5

1

RICE
24-48 hours.

2 **UPPER BODY**
After 48 hours, physiotherapy may now begin, also upper body exercises, sit-ups. Start steps 3, 4, 5.

3 **ISOMETRICS**
Stop hamstring muscle from pulling heel on-to buttocks. Ask someone to hold your leg; or sit and cross ankle of bad leg over front of good ankle. Pull back with bad leg, block movement with good. Hold 7 sec., relax 7 sec., pull 7 sec., repeat 7 times, 3-5 times a day. Isokinetics may start.

4 **STRETCHING**
Use stretching exercises 1, 5, 9, 10, 12 (Chapter 1). Stretch until you feel pain of injury. Hold 15-20 sec. Repeat 3 times. Do sequence 3-5 times a day. Do not bounce. Breathe out to relax.

5 **HEELS**
Facing inward, stand on edge of step with both feet together – do not favour good leg. Raise and lower heels at slow rhythm until calf aches or injury gives pain, then STOP. Repeat 3-5 times during day.

6 **PATTERING AND SKIPPING ROUTINES**

7

SWIMMING ROUTINE

May be omitted if pool, etc., unavailable. Freestyle may hurt. Kick legs gently.

8

BIKE ROUTINE

Do not claw through: to avoid putting strain on injured leg, do NOT drag pedal backward at bottom of its circle by gripping with toes and forefoot and pulling it through the vertical position.

9

ROWING AND BIKE ROUTINES

Bike: OK to claw through. While rowing, coming forward may hurt – work just to discomfort.

10

WEIGHTS

Prone, lying, curls with ankle weights. Curl machine. Isokinetics – pyramid – high speed to low speed and back to high speed. Try one leg bridge: Lie on back with one leg in air, the other bent with foot on ground. Raise hips in air as high as possible; hold – feel hamstring work. Rule of 7. Don't use quads.

11

NO PAIN?

If walking and climbing stairs do not produce pain, move to Hamstring top ladder.

HAMSTRING TOP LADDER

Start each training session from the bottom of the ladder. Early ladder steps may be cut from 6 to 3 repetitions. Continue using Hamstring bottom ladder for fitness. Check that leg rhythm is always equal; do not gallop. One way to avoid favouring injured leg is to count out loud from 1 to 9 while running. This sets rhythm for legs to follow and allows concentration to move from one leg to the other. Counting 1, 2; 1, 2 tends to stress any limp. Do stretching exercises between each 100 yd. (100 m.). Check knee lift and heel pickup are same height. Stop if pain lasts more than 20-30 seconds, or if there is a loss of rhythm.

Start using a ballistic stretch: swing the leg back and forth like a ballet dancer. Because the hamstring decelerates leg ready for impact, it contracts during some stretching. This range is improved by gentle swinging, high ballistic kicks, just to the point of discomfort. As injury improves, build up speed, especially for kicking sports or dancing.

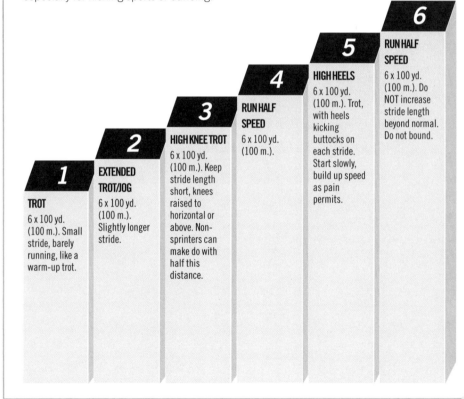

1

TROT

6 x 100 yd. (100 m.). Small stride, barely running, like a warm-up trot.

2

EXTENDED TROT/JOG

6 x 100 yd. (100 m.). Slightly longer stride.

3

HIGH KNEE TROT

6 x 100 yd. (100 m.). Keep stride length short, knees raised to horizontal or above. Non-sprinters can make do with half this distance.

4

RUN HALF SPEED

6 x 100 yd. (100 m.).

5

HIGH HEELS

6 x 100 yd. (100 m.). Trot, with heels kicking buttocks on each stride. Start slowly, build up speed as pain permits.

6

RUN HALF SPEED

6 x 100 yd. (100 m.). Do NOT increase stride length beyond normal. Do not bound.

7

GRADE ONE SPRINT

6 x 100 yd. (100 m.). Accelerate 25 yd. (25 m.); sprint 50 yd. (50 m.); slow down 25 yd. (25 m.).

8

GRADE TWO SPRINT

6 x 100 yd. (100 m.). Accelerate 25 yd. (25 m.); sprint 50 yd. (50 m.); fast stop 25 yd. (25 m.).

Note: Specialist runners should still use slow stop (step 7). Fast stop is only for stop-start sports, usually ball games.

9

GRADE THREE SPRINT

6 x 100 yd. (100 m.). Fast accelerate 25 yd. (25 m.); sprint 50 yd. (50 m.); fast stop 25 yd. (25 m.).

10

SHUTTLE RUN

10 x 20 yd. (20 m.) wind sprints. Sprint back and forth between markers 20 yd. (20 m.) apart.

11

BEANBAG SHUTTLE

As step 10, but incorporate bending to touch or pick up object (such as beanbag) from floor.

12

START PLAY

Begin in easy, low-grade match, easy opposition, until fully fit. Then play at normal grade.

BADMINTON LADDER

This is good for tennis elbow and shoulder injuries.
Find a willing partner who will provide you with the necessary shots. Work 5 minutes at each level. As you move up the ladder, still repeat lower steps as part of training routine. Remember, at the first sign of pain you must stop. If the pain or ache goes away after 20 seconds, continue the exercises. However, if the ache or pain persists – STOP – WAIT 24 hours – begin again from first step. See **How much training to do**. Concentrate grip on 3rd, 4th and 5th fingers. Relax 2nd finger and thumb.

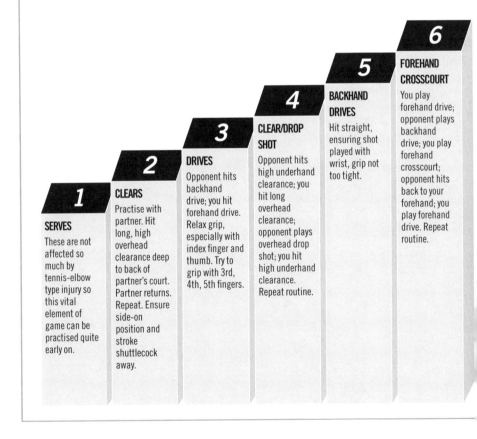

1

SERVES

These are not affected so much by tennis-elbow type injury so this vital element of game can be practised quite early on.

2

CLEARS

Practise with partner. Hit long, high overhead clearance deep to back of partner's court. Partner returns. Repeat. Ensure side-on position and stroke shuttlecock away.

3

DRIVES

Opponent hits backhand drive; you hit forehand drive. Relax grip, especially with index finger and thumb. Try to grip with 3rd, 4th, 5th fingers.

4

CLEAR/DROP SHOT

Opponent hits high underhand clearance; you hit long overhead clearance; opponent plays overhead drop shot; you hit high underhand clearance. Repeat routine.

5

BACKHAND DRIVES

Hit straight, ensuring shot played with wrist, grip not too tight.

6

FOREHAND CROSSCOURT

You play forehand drive; opponent plays backhand drive; you play forehand crosscourt; opponent hits back to your forehand; you play forehand drive. Repeat routine.

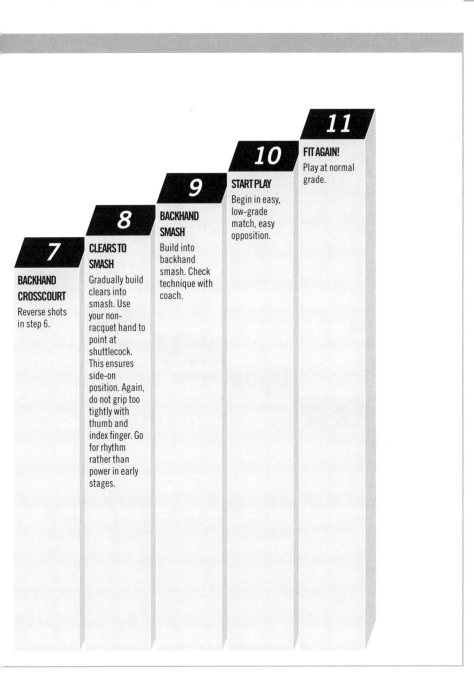

11

FIT AGAIN!

Play at normal grade.

10

START PLAY

Begin in easy, low-grade match, easy opposition.

9

BACKHAND SMASH

Build into backhand smash. Check technique with coach.

8

CLEARS TO SMASH

Gradually build clears into smash. Use your non-racquet hand to point at shuttlecock. This ensures side-on position. Again, do not grip too tightly with thumb and index finger. Go for rhythm rather than power in early stages.

7

BACKHAND CROSSCOURT

Reverse shots in step 6.

TENNIS LADDER

This is good for tennis elbow, which is suffered mainly by those using the standard grip, and single backhand. Semi-Western or Western grip is not often a cause of tennis elbow. If it is, there may be too tight a grip with thumb and 2nd finger.

The Semi-Western grip is most likely to cause golfer's elbow. (Follow steps 1-6, then step 10).

Find a willing partner who will provide you with the necessary shots, or use a tennis machine. Work on technique. Concentrate on footwork and getting sideways onto ball. When playing single-handed backhand, make sure racquet head stays above wrist level; do not lead with elbow. Check with coach if available. Do not snatch at shots. Work 5 minutes at each level. As you move up the ladder repeat lower steps as part of training routine. Remember, at the first sign of pain you must stop. If the pain or ache goes away after 20 seconds, continue the exercises. However, if the ache or pain persists – STOP – WAIT 24 hours – begin again from first step. Do not grip racquet too tightly with thumb and index finger.

STANDARD GRIP

1	2	3	4	5	6
FOREHAND FLAT	FOREHAND TOPSPIN	FOREHAND VOLLEY	SECOND SERVE	FIRST SERVE	FLAT SERVICE / Go for rhythm not power.

SEMI-WESTERN GRIP

BACKHAND	VOLLEYS	STROKED FOREHAND	BACKHAND FLAT	BACKHAND VOLLEY	WHIPPED FOREHAND / Now move to level 10. of the standard grip ladder.

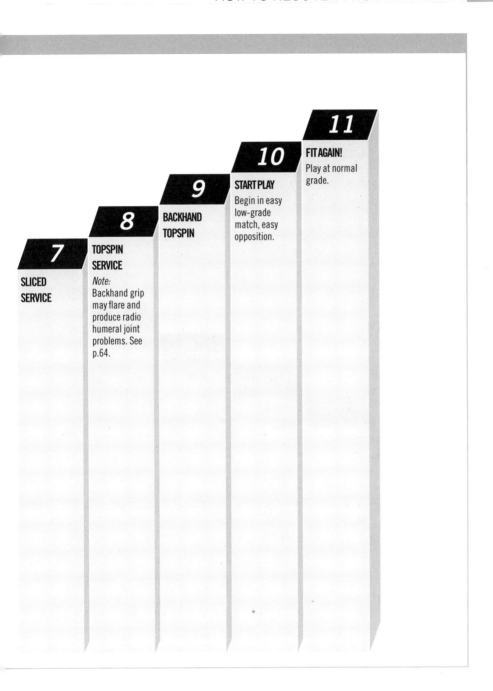

11

FIT AGAIN!
Play at normal grade.

10

START PLAY
Begin in easy low-grade match, easy opposition.

9

BACKHAND TOPSPIN

8

TOPSPIN SERVICE
Note:
Backhand grip may flare and produce radio humeral joint problems. See p.64.

7

SLICED SERVICE

SQUASH LADDER

Useful for most injuries since, as you will know where the ball is going, you will not be wrong-footed. For golfer's elbow problems, use the steps in a different order as follows: 1, 4, 7, 2, 6, 5, 3, 8, 9, 10.

Find a willing partner who will provide you with the necessary shots. Work 5 minutes at each level. As you move up the ladder, repeat lower steps as part of training routine. Remember, at the first sign of pain you must stop. If the pain or ache goes away after 20 seconds, continue the exercises. However, if the ache or pain persists – STOP – WAIT 24 hours – begin again from first step.

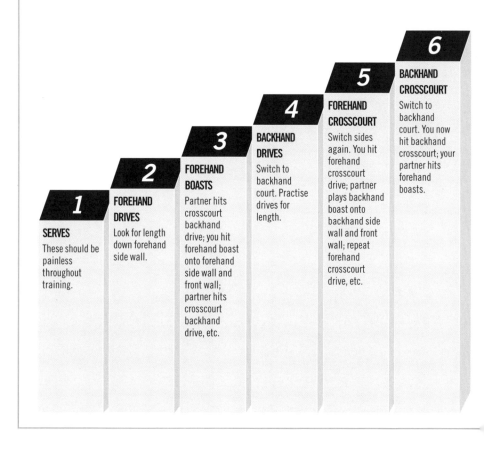

1

SERVES

These should be painless throughout training.

2

FOREHAND DRIVES

Look for length down forehand side wall.

3

FOREHAND BOASTS

Partner hits crosscourt backhand drive; you hit forehand boast onto forehand side wall and front wall; partner hits crosscourt backhand drive, etc.

4

BACKHAND DRIVES

Switch to backhand court. Practise drives for length.

5

FOREHAND CROSSCOURT

Switch sides again. You hit forehand crosscourt drive; partner plays backhand boast onto backhand side wall and front wall; repeat forehand crosscourt drive, etc.

6

BACKHAND CROSSCOURT

Switch to backhand court. You now hit backhand crosscourt; your partner hits forehand boasts.

7 BACKHAND BOASTS

You play backhand boasts; your partner plays forehand crosscourt.

8 PAIRED, AND BOAST AND DRIVE

You hit forehand boast, partner hits straight backhand drive. You hit backhand boast; partner hits straight forehand drive. Swap position with partner and reverse play.

9 SMASH

Concentrate on holding racquet with 3rd, 4th and 5th fingers rather than thumb and index finger. Try to avoid face on position.

10 PLAY GAME

Use special rules. Insist there should be no drop shots, that ball must bounce over half-court line, but hard drive, bouncing shorter, permitted.

11 START PLAY

Begin in easy, low-grade match, easy opposition.

12 FIT AGAIN!

Play at normal grade.

BASEBALL LADDER

Find a willing partner. Work 5 minutes at each level. As you move up the ladder, repeat lower steps as part of training routine. Remember, at the first sign of pain you must stop. If the pain or ache goes away after 20 seconds, continue the exercises. However, if the ache or pain persists – STOP – WAIT 24 hours – begin again from first step. The shoulder muscles must build up strength not only to throw but also to stop the shoulders following the ball! Observe principles of training as it is easy to overdo this ladder.

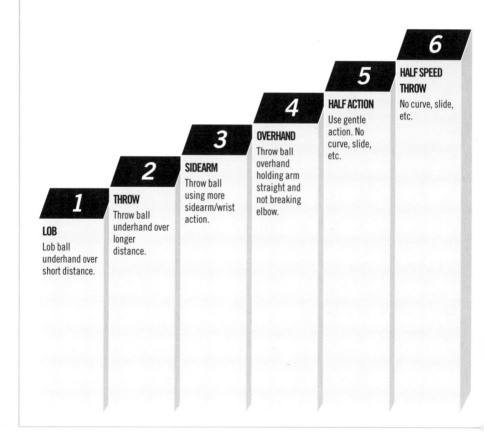

1

LOB

Lob ball underhand over short distance.

2

THROW

Throw ball underhand over longer distance.

3

SIDEARM

Throw ball using more sidearm/wrist action.

4

OVERHAND

Throw ball overhand holding arm straight and not breaking elbow.

5

HALF ACTION

Use gentle action. No curve, slide, etc.

6

HALF SPEED THROW

No curve, slide, etc.

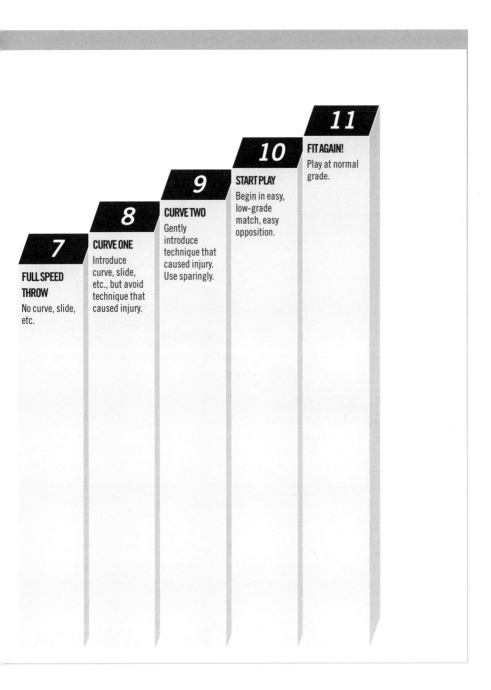

7

FULL SPEED THROW

No curve, slide, etc.

8

CURVE ONE

Introduce curve, slide, etc., but avoid technique that caused injury.

9

CURVE TWO

Gently introduce technique that caused injury. Use sparingly.

10

START PLAY

Begin in easy, low-grade match, easy opposition.

11

FIT AGAIN!

Play at normal grade.

Home and Workplace

Back and neck

The back and neck cause most problems whether you are sitting at a desk or bending over garden or household task. Many of these problems can be avoided if you observe the following:

• Do not wedge the telephone between head and shoulder as this twists the neck sideways producing facet and disc problems. Use shoulder holster or headset.

• Adjust computer and chair to the correct height. If the computer terminal is set too low on the desk and the chair too high, or if you wear bifocals, you may sit slumped with a rounded back, hyperextending the neck for long periods during the day.

• The computer screen should be about 15-30° down from the head position, and the keyboard and mouse operated with relaxed shoulders and bent elbows. If the screen and keyboard are offset from centre, then upper back problems will join neck problems. Most people sit too slumped over a long day and the lower and upper back need to be straightened so that the head is balanced – not looking up or down and not pushed forward.

• Office chairs should be fully adjustable – the tilt of the seat, the back and the height should all be adjustable to each individual user.

• Try a kneel-on chair or use seat wedges (thinner at the front) and lumbar rolls, if your back pain is worse while sitting and especially if it is eased by stretching backward when you stand up after sitting.

NOTE

Lumbar supports in a chair are useless unless they adjust up and down to fit the hollow in your back (as opposed to that of someone taller or shorter than you).

• If no seat adjustments are available, try to sit at the front of the chair (sideways on a sofa) and point one knee towards the ground. Drop the knee far enough to comfortably straighten your back.

• Car seats, despite all the adjustments available, often leave the arms too far from the steering wheel and the head against the roof. Those with back problems need to sit nearer the steering wheel with bent arms in order to take the tension out of back and sit taller. It is worth looking for a car that suits your back.

• No one goes out and runs for 2-3 hours without any training, yet people will go into the garden and do 2 hours of weeding and digging and wonder why they have back problems. Learn to bend with a neutral to arched (hollowed) back, buttocks out, hip and knees bent, weight over middle of feet. (See p. 79.)

• Plan 5-10 minutes of bending jobs round the house and garden followed by 5-10 minutes of standing/reaching jobs and continue in this fashion.

• Try vacuuming to your side and slightly behind you.

• Standing half-bent over a sink, ironing board, etc. is a killer for the back. Stand

with legs wide apart – this drops your height without bending your back or straining your knees. Lean the front of your thighs into the side of the sink and hold a neutral back, which will enable you to lean and reach into the sink.
• Use the bottom-out back position for all half-bent positions – from brushing teeth to making the bed, to emptying the car or oven.

Elbow and shoulder
Tennis elbow can interfere with many activities.
• Thicken your pen with tape and try holding between second and third fingers or relax tight pinch grip.
• Don't hold computer mouse too tightly
• Lift office files, briefcase, etc. palm upward until better.
• Use screwdrivers with long handles or those that are power driven; use a mechanical whisk.
• Avoid hammering, long pruning sessions or operating a hedge trimmer above shoulder height, all of which will make tennis elbow flare.
• Be careful digging, trowelling, weeding and pulling out plants as this can produce golfer's elbow.
• Leaning an elbow on the windowsill, etc. may compress the ulnar nerve or funnybone.

Shoulder problems are usually impingement or rotator cuff caused by working too long above shoulder height with paintbrush, hedge trimmers etc.
• Climb as high as possible when cleaning so that you can work mainly

below shoulder height. Remember that reaching out over a table or under furniture to polish also takes your arms above your shoulders.
• Stretching your hand span wide – especially the thumb – when polishing or opening jars may, for example, flare De Quervain of thumb and wrist.

Knee
Be aware of the following:
• Some office workers wrap their legs around the chair, or cross their knees, then wrap one foot under the other ankle. These contortions can produce ligament sprains of the knee or pins and needles and numbness from the peroneal nerve.
• Use a polystyrene or sheepskin pad if you have to do a lot of kneeling to avoid calluses and housemaid's knee (prepatellar bursa).
• Ankle, hip and knee injuries can be helped by balancing on one leg while on the telephone, waiting for a bus, etc.
• Many knee problems are helped by walking slowly down the stairs, with control. For tracking knee problems, you must keep the knee vertical above the foot when going upstairs.

5

Sport-by-Sport Guide to Technical Injuries

Every sport in the world makes different demands on the participants and their bodies. Some require endurance; others speed. Some need great flexibility; others great technical skill.

Although there are many injuries that are common to many sports, some problems are specific to certain sports. Using this sport-by-sport rundown, you can spot the peculiarities of your own particular sport and be better prepared to avoid injuries – or to recognize them if you or your team-mates are unlucky enough to suffer them.

Injuries that have already been explained in the Top-to-Toe Guide (Chapter 3) are in bold face.

Injuries such as Quads expansion, Lower patella pole, Jumper's knee and Osgood Schlatter's disease are all caused by too much training or too much power being applied to mechanisms such as the knee. These are referred to as overload injuries. Patella pain, Plica, Patella facet pain are caused by the kneecap not moving properly in the thighbone (femur) grooves and are referred to as tracking problems. The fault may be caused by the foot, knee or hip.

Archery

Archers are not prone to serious injuries, but can avoid annoying ones by using equipment tailored to their needs. The bow must, of course, be the correct weight because too heavy a draw-weight (bow weight) can be tiring and can produce overuse muscle injuries in the upper body and arms. Finger tabs should suit the individual.

Tennis elbow can occur in the arm holding the bow when the wrist is extended through the draw before locking it into the support position. Although this may help the draw, it could mean the draw-weight is too heavy.

Biceps strain from using too heavy a draw-weight heals after a proper rest but suggests that the shoulder blade muscles are not being used to draw. Check technique with coach and resume training with a lighter bow.

Badminton

At the very top level, this is one of the most physically demanding sports. Footwear is important as many matches are played on firm, composition floors rather than sprung wooden surfaces. Properly padded shoes absorb shock and help prevent blisters and forefoot strains, but the soles should not be as thick or high as trainers as they become unstable for this quick change-of-direction sport. The knee on the racquet-hand side is susceptible to great stresses, both overload and tracking. Although pain is common in the wrists and shoulders, this is often due to poor footwork. Striking the shuttle when in an awkward, off-balance position strains the joints. Correct technique not only makes shots more effective, but also avoids injury.

A/C joint injury could ruin a season since overhead shots cause the condition to flare up. As below-the-shoulder shots are pain free, try squash during the lay-off period and seek medical advice.

Painful arc/rotator cuff or **subacromial joint injuries** need to be diagnosed accurately if the technical fault is to be corrected. They are caused by hitting too hard with the shoulder or smashing from too far behind the head; the best way to treat them is to reduce the power of the shot and hit with the wrist. Check with a coach that you are not smashing face on and that your feet are correctly positioned. Early cortisone injections are of value, and in severe cases, fitness can be maintained by playing squash.

Tennis elbow is common, especially in doubles, where the net player has to angle forehand interceptions. If the grip is too tight (using the thumb and index finger), the wrist is not released enough to angle the shot, so the elbow is jammed straight, flaring the radio-humeral joint. Check your grip and technique with a coach; try a thicker grip and hold with the 3rd, 4th and 5th fingers. Another cause of tennis elbow is the tendency to come face on to the smash, before whipping the shot with the wrist. See Badminton ladder plan.

Incorrect lunging can cause severe lower back, hamstring and Achilles tendon problems. Stretching and strengthening of these areas is important to minimize problems. Sufferers from **adductor muscle strain** should avoid overstretching sideways when building back into competition; extra coaching on

footwork is required. The "round the head" shot may inflame the sartorius muscle. See **Unstable knee** and **Rapid swelling** and seek early medical advice.

A pull-off fracture of the thigh is produced by repeated lunging, which loads the quads; this is common in growing youngsters. Seek medical advice. Players suffering from quads overload should avoid reaching over the knee during training to pick up drop shots. Only play shuttlecock above the waist until pain free and reduce quads training; build via doubles to singles.

Impingement injuries of the ankle occur in the trail leg from deep lunging, so check footwork. Turn trail foot out sideways (as fencers do) rather than lunge over a toes-forward straight foot. **Plantar fasciitis** is common on non-sprung floors, and even half-rising on the toes when preparing to smash may hurt. Heel cups, shock-absorbing wedges and strapping may help – check heel cup of shoe is stable. Concentrate on pattering for fitness while running is painful.

Baseball/Softball

Baseball players rarely look as fit as they could and should be. In a game involving sudden moves after long periods of inactivity, hamstrings are likely to go in the sprint for first base, while groin pulls occur in attempting awkward ground balls. Thorough warm-ups and stretching are vital.

The most publicized injury is **pitcher's elbow**, which covers a multitude of sins caused by slightly different techniques and throws. Fast snapping of the elbow into extension, especially if the wrist cock is maintained throughout delivery as in the change-up and fastball, causes **olecranon fossa, olecranon fracture** and **triceps strain. A radio-humeral joint sprain** can be flared by pitching the screwball, so avoid overusing this delivery if it is causing problems. **Golfer's elbow**, a type of pitcher's elbow, is an overuse injury, caused by trying to gain more speed on the fastball by pitching the curveball or slider. Both release the cocked wrist through delivery, and three-quarter action increases the risk.

Little league elbow/pull-off fracture is the same injury in a growing child. One of the problems of the sport is over-enthusiastic youngsters (or worse, youngsters encouraged by over-enthusiastic parents) damaging themselves by repeatedly throwing fastballs. It is possible that the three-quarter action (more common in beginners) plays a part. As the bones are still growing, any elbow injury must be treated seriously and examined by a medical expert. There is the risk that growth may be permanently impaired. Most pitching by youngsters is supervised to control the number of pitches per week, and many coaches forbid the throwing of curveballs. A diary to record the number of pitches each week is essential and should not be abused by sneaking in extra practice sessions. Technique, accuracy and control should be encouraged rather than speed. As soon as a youngster says, "It hurts when I throw", stop play, seek medical advice.

If throwing is painless sidearm but painful overarm, chances are that it is a **shoulder separation/A/C joint injury** if there has been a shoulder problem from a fall or from sliding into base. **Shoulder impingement/subacromial bursa** injury can occur when fielders attempt to throw too hard overarm. Throw side- or underarm. Treat early with cortisone injections. Underlying **rotator cuff** damage or weakness will need specific rehabilitation as these muscles not only generate power and control shoulder position, but also stop the arm following the ball. Most shoulder work developed in gyms does not strengthen these rotator cuff muscles. Consult a qualified fitness coach. Good lower body strength can help the upper body by taking some of the strain off the arm through proper take-off and follow through.

Jammed fingers are common. See a doctor if they are out of line. Tape a jammed finger to a healthy one for support. **Mallet or baseball finger** is more serious, as the tip of the finger droops and cannot be straightened. This needs splinting by a doctor.

Techniques for sliding into base are important, but few agree on a correct method. Putting the full weight of the body at speed onto an ankle that is resisted by a rough surface is asking for trouble. One school of thought suggests sliding head first into second and third base. As the catcher is a pretty solid object, feet first is advisable at home plate. Whether your coach accepts this or not, everyone agrees that indecision is the worst decision!

Basketball/Handball/Netball/Volleyball

All involve jumping, twisting and turning so ligament injuries are common, particularly when one player is liable to land on another player's foot. Some experts argue that braced or taped ankles will increase the torque on the knee joint, but recent evidence suggests that preventive bracing of the ankle does cut down the overall number of injuries. Lace-up ankle braces save time and money compared with conventional taping and are as effective.

As the hands have to deal with a large ball, **mallet finger**, **sprained thumb** and **dislocated finger** injuries are inherent problems, so strapping the joints is both beneficial and preventive. Feet, knees and ankles are a problem when these sports are played on firm surfaces, so footwear must be well padded to reduce risk from jumping and landing, checking and changing direction.

Rapid checking and explosive jumping both produce knee overload injuries. During rehabilitation, practise stationary throws, building into lay-ups as the pain settles. However, if pain starts again during practice then you should stop. Return to static shooting to avoid any delay to healing.

All these games, which involve twisting side to side can produce **adductor strains** and **footballer's groin** (conjoined tendon). If your adductor muscle is not settling, seek experienced medical advice. **Jumper's leg** is an overload problem but a persistent **jumper's ankle** may be due to a small bone (os trigonum) which causes problems in these sports and may need surgery.

Handballers are particularly susceptible to shoulder-throwing injuries such as **shoulder impingement** (**subacromial bursa**), **painful arc** (**rotator cuff**) and, following falls, **shoulder separation/A/C joint**.

Bowling

Scarcely the most energetic sport, it still produces some peculiar afflictions, such as **bowler's elbow**, a strain of the elbow joint, from the sheer weight of the ball. RICE is advised. Check the weight and correct drilling of holes in a personalized ball if you are a frequent participant as the ligaments of the fingers (particularly 3rd and 4th) may be sprained. Thumb irritation and calluses are common among regular bowlers. Cover sore areas and sand down calluses. Trying to increase the spin on the ball may cause the whole arm to finish across and in front of the body, straining the shoulder. Even the sheer weight of transporting half a dozen competition balls around can cause shoulder and elbow problems. Bowler's toe afflicts as many as a third of all bowlers due to the stress placed on the big and second toes of the trailing foot on delivery. Check footwear to avoid misshapen toes, thickened toenails and calluses.

Bowls

Another gentle sport, where only the onset of old age, together with arthritis, dictates a change of technique. Concentration on the neutral back position on delivery will prevent further problems.

Boxing

Apart from the obvious pummelling that the head, hands and upper body take, there is damage peculiar to the sport such as **cut eyes**. Dilute adrenalin may be used during the bout, but it is essential that early pressure and ice are applied and (if needed) sutures rather than adhesive stitches to give the best results. The suturing (stitching) should be under the skin, with great care being taken to approximate the edges of the wound. Enzyme creams minimize scarring, but 3 weeks are needed for skin to regain its normal strength, even if it appears to be healed much sooner, so always use head guards for sparring. If a boxer is shortsighted he should be aware that there is a proven connection between high myopia and an increased likelihood of a detached retina. Laser correction does not alter this risk.

Some boxers may develop a congenital spur of bone in the muscle tendon just above the elbow. A direct blow can break it off, causing **boxer's arm**, a pain in the upper arm. Hands, especially the metacarpals, may suffer fractures or subluxation.

Do not dehydrate for fights to "make the weight". A 5 per cent weight loss by dehydration causes a 20-30 per cent drop in work rate; accelerated fatigue causes loss of head and neck control, so a punch to the head can rotate the brain. Neck muscles always require strength work. After a **Knockout/KO**, amateur boxers are not allowed to fight again for 28 days (first time), 84 days (second time) and one year (third time). The risk is punch drunkenness (brain damage), and regular brain (CT or MRI) scans are now part of professional boxing.

Canoeing and Kayaking

Basic safety drill must always be understood, even by the best swimmers. Hypothermia (see Chapter 1 Some Sensible Tips) is a risk: Be prepared. Although wildwater paddlers know about the risks, leisure paddlers often forget how cold paddle splashes can be. Use a body wetsuit (low cut under arms, loose rubber/plastic sleeves) in cold conditions, even when training or on holiday.

Paddler's wrist (De Quervain) is common in kayakers, who feel pain on the lower end of the forearm when extending the wrist and hand in a claw position (as if paddling or rowing). **Biceps tendinitis** can also occur, more often in the shoulder than the elbow, due to overuse because of pulling too much on one arm without pushing with the other. Check with a coach in case your pull/twist technique is faulty because some specially shaped paddles may ease the problem. **Tennis elbow** is often caused by lack of forearm strength to take strain as well as faulty technique. Consult a coach.

Many aches and pains can be corrected by checking the width of your grip (upper body strains) and placement of the seat in relation to the footrest/rudder control (lower neutral backs). A twisting strain on the back is likely to flare upper back pain, so seek manipulation early. Hunching up to generate more power overloads the midback, so make sure the neutral back position is second nature before increasing paddling thrust.

Novice canoeists can suffer **housemaid's knee** from kneeling, or calluses on the bones one sits on (ischeal tuberosity), so use a polystyrene pad lined with sheepskin as protection and give the knee a chance to adapt by short and frequent training sessions early on.

Cricket

The apparent lack of athleticism in cricketers is matched only by that of baseball players, but the better sides have a sensible attitude to stretching and fitness. Over a long day, dehydration can lessen a player's effectiveness. (See: Dehydration, p. 16). Although concentration over hours can be helped by chewing gum, a number of batsmen have inhaled gum and nearly died.

Apart from the obvious dangers and discomforts threatened by the use of a hard ball for which increasing protective armour is used, cricketers suffer shoulder, back and knee problems. **A/C joint strain** is a classic example of an injury that prevents overarm bowling or throwing, though side and underarm efforts are pain free. Hard throws from the boundary reflare the injury, so either field closer or be satisfied with threatening a hard throw – and then return underarm. Cortisone injections may be required.

With the **subacromial bursa**, the overarm bowling action is painless, but hard overarm throws hurt. Treat with cortisone injections and throw in sidearm or underarm. Off-season throwing drills and rotator cuff strengthening are essential.

Any catching sport, especially with a hard ball, risks **fractured, dislocated** and **mallet fingers**.

Bowlers' backs suffer, and this is usually from the facet joints. **Bowler's back**, however, is a stress fracture with pain on the opposite side of the bowling arm and worse in extension. Bowling action should be front on or side on, but a mixed action is most likely to cause this stress fracture. Check with coach. Some limit, such as a bowling diary, should be placed on children and young cricketers to reduce the number of fast balls bowled.

Overload knee problems are common in close fielders but usually occur (for right-arm bowlers) in the left leg at delivery. **Lower patella pole** is more common with inswing bowlers, who are balanced on the left knee for a fraction longer on delivery. The answer could be to cut down on speed and concentrate on away swingers until pain free.

The quick single played to the leg off the back foot may induce calf or Achilles problems. Stress fractures occur in the shins of many bowlers. Reduction in pace and number of deliveries plus mechanical correction is the only effective treatment.

Cycling

The bicycle itself governs many of the

aches and pains suffered by cyclists, and correct fitting of frame size is essential.

The pedal arcs, saddle and handlebars can be adjusted, so that anyone of any size can have a proper fit.

• Saddle to the handlebars: Use your forearm to measure this. With your elbow touching the front of the saddle, your outstretched fingers should touch the midpoint of the handlebars. A low back pain from a creeping disc is not uncommon. Try to keep the back less bowed, lengthen frame or use tribars to flatten and obtain neutral back position.

• Saddle height: To find the correct height, sit on the saddle with your leg straight (not stretched). Your heel should be on the pedal, with the pedal at its lowest point.

• Handlebar height: The handlebars should be level with the saddle. If you are not comfortable even after the adjustments, you may have too small or too big a bicycle. If a frame is too small or the handlebars too low, this can cause compression or "springing" over the lower ribs. A coach can work out a better position.

As riders lean forward in the racing position, acid can tip out of the stomach causing heartburn. Stomach gas can press on the diaphragm, so take antacids (or oil of peppermint on a sugar lump) before races.

Aches and pains occur in the bottom, because of a poorly positioned saddle or even tight, uncomfortable clothing. Boils are common if dirty clothing is worn or if a body hair has grown back into the skin, causing infection.

Long-distance riders have unusual problems, confined only to cycling, including a numb penis or persistent erection. This is due to pressure on certain nerves or veins and should be reported to a doctor if the condition persists once a saddle adjustment has been made.

Hand pain often occurs in novices, but gloves and padded handlebars help. Beware numbness in the 4th and little fingers as this means the **ulnar nerve** is being pinched. Numbness in the thumb, 1st and 2nd fingers could be **Carpal tunnel syndrome**. Check grip on handlebar.

Knees and ankles suffer from overuse in a sport that demands riders put "miles in their legs". The only sensible solution is to cycle using easier gears and reduce mileage, building back up slowly to high gears. Avoid climbing hills until high gears on the flat are pain free. Tracking problems can occur at the knee, especially if knees do not stay vertically in line over the feet. Raising the saddle may help – but check forefoot with orthotics expert as wedge in shoe may rebalance foot. Clip-on toe catch must have "play" within it as totally fixed foot can stop natural compensation.

Darts
Youngsters who want to emulate the professionals might decide to spend 3 or 4 hours practising. The result of this sudden exertion is **dart thrower's elbow**, which is technically **olecranon bursa**. The other hazard is dartitis, where a player gets the equivalent of writer's cramp and

just cannot release the dart. This can be as much psychological as physical.

Diving and Trampolining

Diving headfirst into water is the commonest cause of para- and tetraplegias. If you do not know the depth of the water or whether obstacles exist, always slide into the water feet-first.

Divers are usually carefully coached, graduating from exercise to exercise. There are relatively few impact injuries from hitting the board or breaking the fingers on reverse or inward dives; even more rare are head injuries from spinning above the board and hitting it coming down. Blood on the board should be cleaned with bleach or antiseptic. The dilutional factor as well as the chlorine in the pool should eliminate any danger of infection to others. More frequent are strains and sprains of the hand, thumb, wrist, shoulders and neck in highboard diving, where divers hit the water repeatedly at 60 mph (100 kph). neutral back from piked one-and-a-half somersaults is common, due to the twist movement and arching of the back, while beginners may get facet pains from being forced into hyperextension. Manipulation may help. Some incidence of **Osgood Schlatter's disease** has been noted amongst young divers on take off or "springing" the board too frequently.

Trampolining certainly looks like great fun but must be supervised at all times. Surprisingly, a large number of injuries are suffered in folding and unfolding the powerful, spring-loaded beds. This is not a job for children.

Painful joint instability (ankle and knee) is common, and many accidents among youngsters occur due to the G (gravity) forces exerted that make them black out for a moment, lose control and land awkwardly. In spite of an emphasis on safety, there are still a worrying number of accidents in the sport, and medical experts in many countries recommend that trampolining should not be a school sport because of the inherent competitiveness that it often encourages. Awkward neck injuries may cause tetraplegia, so catchers should be on duty at all four sides of the trampoline. Worn equipment, especially at beaches, etc., is very dangerous. The rebound from the trampoline can produce overload knee problems. See: Head warning (p. 42).

Equestrian sports

Most injuries are from bites, kicks and falls. Falls produce most of the injuries and should be dealt with by first-aid principles. Always take special care with neck injuries. Those involved in riding horses should take first-aid courses. Point-to-point racing with its enthusiastic amateurs and highly trained horses has a very high severe injury and death rate (See: Head warning, p. 42). As thigh strength is so important, training the quads muscles while off the horse is invaluable, but tracking knee problems may prove particularly troublesome for those wanting to ride competitively and will need medical help. **Adductor muscle strains** and acute tears can occur when jumping. Any technical faults can lead to strains and, if they unbalance the horse, result in falls and poor dressage. It is particularly important when the rider is recovering from an injury not to rush back onto the horse. Get yourself fully fit again or take the consequences of unbalancing the horse.

Fencing

The sport is deceptive as endurance, strength and flexibility are all required to get to the top. Equipment must be checked frequently (especially masks) because any defect can result in injury. However blunt a sword may look, the lunging force behind it is considerable, and penetration of a face mask can be fatal. Look for signs of rusting on your face mask (caused by regularly breathing on it) and always strap on gear properly. If you are an occasional fencer, lower the risk of injury by stretching properly. In competition, repeated bouts are tiring because fencing suits promote high fluid loss. High glucose fluids, special fluid energy drinks or plain water will maintain fluid balance and blood sugar levels and put off fatigue.

Football, American

This is a sport where size and speed are the dominant factors. It is vital to learn the correct way to block and tackle or else risk an injury. A big, powerful runner may well cause injuries purely because at the school, even college, level, there is an inequality of size. Awkward falls are almost inevitable. Ligament sprains result from twisting, sidestepping movements. Using knee braces to prevent injury does not seem as successful as wearing braces on the ankles.

Major improvements in helmet design give more protection, while supportive collars have reduced neck injuries. Because size and strength are so important, many injuries are triggered in the gym due to over-enthusiasm in training, producing overuse injuries from excessive weight training.

Training and playing on artificial turf may cause **black toe/turf toe**. Try putting padding along the sides of the big toe or tongue of the shoe to hold the width of the foot more firmly and so prevent it from driving into the toe of the shoe when stopping suddenly.

Some injuries have names like "halfback hamstring," but this is not specific to the sport. As in rugby, baseball, etc., where players may stand idle for periods and then suddenly have to sprint into action, the hamstring is always likely to suffer if not kept stretched and warm.

Jersey finger is common to other sports too. A quick grab at a player as he rushes by can result in a painful tweak (even **mallet finger**) to the top joint of the finger. Adductor strains that do not settle may be **footballer's groin (conjoined tendon)**, which requires experienced medical advice. Falls on the shoulder often cause **shoulder separation** or **A/C joint disruption** and **shoulder dislocation** can occur in tackles.

Golf

Golfers fall into two general groups: those

that learn golf as youngsters and those that have taken up the game as a second or retirement sport. Golfing aches and pains are also split into two categories. Some problems, such as arthritis, back pain and aching feet, have nothing to do with the way the game is played. The rest of the problems are often due to poor technique.

The obvious problem of golf, especially at a later age, is unaccustomed walking. Collapsed arches, bunions and so on may be helped by appropriate orthotics for the shoes. These may also help **arthritis of the knee**, as will lightweight thigh muscle work. **Arthritis of the hip** and a stiff spine need regular loose swings of the hands and arms, often with an open stance. Back sufferers should work on a "sit down" stance. When teeing up or picking the ball out of the hole, bend down on one leg, holding the other straight out behind with toe on ground. Use neutral back/bottom-out position to pick up your golfbag; pull your trolley with a hand-under/palm-up grip. Neck problems will also limit rotation, so just accept the arms doing more.

Golf is a highly technical sport, producing a wide range of nagging, technical injuries. If a problem persists, consult an expert. Problems actually caused by golf can depend on the level of play. The following descriptions are all for right-handers.

Good players: Suffer mainly low back problems from extension of right side under the shot into the follow through. Often **facet joint** – freeing up manipulation may help. Sacroiliac joint

and facets on right side are overloaded by increasing the coil tension in the legs on the take away. **Golfer's elbow** is thought to be from sheer power with the right arm through the shot with a longish divot and **tennis elbow** from too tight a thumb and index finger grip, while an attempt to force the thumb down the shaft can produce **De Quervain**. Sometimes just a thicker grip will help to overcome these problems. Lumbar disc problems may came from spending a long time half bent over – a longer handle may help. **Ulnar nerve pain** and pisihamate ligament problems can occur from the club handle, especially if shot blocked by heavy rough, etc.

Not-so-good players: The contortions adopted both at the address and through the swing are legion and many will produce aches and strains – often a good sports medicine doctor can diagnose your golf fault by the muscle that hurts! Perhaps golfing-great Henry Cotton's training method of just standing up and hitting an old car tire with the club would give us all our most natural swing. Below are some clues to the area of pain/discomfort and then the possible cause:

• Left calf or achilles: Reverse pivot over bent knee with raised heel.
• Left inside knee, cartilage ligaments: Reverse pivot, over bent knee keeping heel on ground.
• Right inside knee, cartilage ligaments : Falling back on shot, probably from reverse pivot.
• Low back: Too bowed over shot, or a rigid right leg at take away.

- Upper back: Overswinging.
- Right **shoulder impingement** (**subacromial bursa**): Flying right elbow on take away.
- Left rotator cuff: Left side pushed forward and tense at the address; arm take away; no shoulder rotation.
- Left tennis elbow: High hands and wrists at address make hands break away early on take away.
- Right tennis elbow: Closed right-hand grip forces you to release thumb and index finger at top of swing.
- Shoulder blade rub: Hunched back, rigid straight arm at address.
- Rib pain: This could be due to stress fractures. Consult doctor.

Gymnastics

Competitors receives scores out of 10. Techniques are continuously repeated by youngsters, so overuse injuries are almost inevitable. Despite the popularity of the sport, not everyone has the right physique for it. Medical advice should therefore be heeded when it comes to **swayback elbow** for example.

Swayback elbow or hyperextension is caused when the elbow is straightened too far. There is acute pain in the joint. The injury is common as competitors spend as much time on their hands as their feet. While the normal elbow can go 5 or 10 degrees beyond 180, the swayback elbow goes back even further, straining the ligaments that hold the upper and lower arm bones together. Complete rest is essential, although muscle-stretching exercises may be continued for shoulders and legs.

Youngsters who aim to take part in Olympic-style gymnastics, and who have swayback elbows or hypermobile joints, are strongly advised to consider switching to another type of sport, perhaps rhythmic gymnastics. Repeated injuries destroy confidence, technical faults develop in an effort to get around the problem, with the result that complex moves can become dangerous.

The wrist also takes a lot of stress, purely from extension in the handstand position. Wrist braces may not help but padding the butt of the palm reduces wrist extension as does turning the hands so that the fingers point outward instead of forward. A **stress fracture** of the growing point of the radius tends to occur in the fulcral or pivotal wrist when doing twisting vaults, but the constant repetition needed to practise floor work may also contribute. Certainly those starting out on the pommel horse may find that both wrists are sore. Although all training that hurts the wrist must be avoided, work on the beam and bars should be all right in the earliest stages of rehabilitating the injury. Maintain stretching, and after about four weeks, when weight can be taken on the wrist without pain, handstands can be tried. Using the ladder principles (see Chapter 4), graduate to walkovers (no flic-flacs, somersaults) and when healed, graduate via straight vaults, flic-flacs, somersaults to twisting vaults. Avoid heavy-twisting vault sessions; preferably, alternate with other routines every other day. Check with a doctor on balancing progress with training.

There are three main causes for **gymnast's back**.

1 When a youngster tries to achieve too much too soon, hyperextension of the back is concentrated on one spot. Correct this by increasing shoulder mobility and train extension of the spine to be spread all down the lower spine in a smooth arch rather than an acute angle.
2 Overworking the trail leg in backward walkovers and the lead leg in forward walkovers is second cause. Try alternating lead legs, even if this is difficult, and lengthening the arc of the circle. Rest if necessary.
3 The most important cause is stress fracture of the spine, spondylolysis (see: Bowler's back, Gymnast's back). This is caused from extension under impact and/or rotation. Persistent pain should be checked by either SPECT scan, MRI or CT scan. Training should reduce extension and impaction, but note grand circles on rings can produce a whiplash extension with the same result.

The force of landing hard after a dismount (over-rotating forward, under-rotating backward) can cause quadriceps and knee overload. When too painful to land, do no vaults or dismounts or use landing pit. Work on the bars, the beam (without squat) and check on the mat that walkovers are trouble free. If pain on run up and take off, do floor suppling and arm balance and build to walkovers as the condition improves. Then, using the ladder system, build up via vaulting pit, rolled landings to spot landings. Try to avoid heavy floor and vault training on the same day – do alternate days of floor and bar; vault and beam. Impingement injury to ankle can also be caused by over-rotating forward and under-rotating backward on landing. Roll out of landings until better; save spot landings for competition. Correct the technical fault.

There are obvious, visible injuries from falls, and in men's gymnastics, where arm strength is everything, the shoulders suffer. Large protective calluses are also characteristic of the sport (see: A-Z of Common ailments, p. 32).

Handball
See: Basketball.

Hockey, Field
The widespread use of artificial turf and the growth of indoor hockey has produced new injuries in a game characterized by the need to run in a bent position over the stick. This results in **high knee hip**, which flares up after long and unaccustomed training sessions, especially if dribbling the ball. Artificial surfaces increase the driving style of running with the ball on the open stick. It is necessary to build up gradually to this style and vary training sessions to allow rest.

Footballer's groin occurs in hockey, especially on hard or artificial surfaces where defenders back off, twisting from side to side. Knee overload has been increased by the low tackling position and when the stick-stopper traps the ball during excessive practice sessions for short corner drills. Have short, sharp sessions rather than long ones.

Jumper's ankle occurs in hockey in the left foot of players (especially left-wingers at speed) who stamp hard before a reverse stick check. Switch position until healed or use a shorter running stride.

Black toe/Turf toe is common on dry, artificial turf when a sudden stop drives the toe into the front of the shoe. As the sport has developed into a year-round game, **teenager's knee** is more common. Any swelling in a youngster's knee, when there has been no fall, must be treated seriously.

Veterans often suffer **hamstring injuries** due to lack of suppleness as they run and bend to collect a ball or to tackle, so they should maintain stretching and fitness. Blows on the hands are common. RICE bruises as soon as possible, but check for fractures. With the added pace when shooting the ball on hard and artificial surfaces, goalkeepers must always wear the correct face and body protection.

Horse riding
See: Equestrian sports.

Jogging
See: Track and Field Athletics.

Judo
In this highly disciplined sport, players learn techniques under supervision and are only matched against players of similar ability and size. Falling and throwing properly are taught from the start. Although requiring great strength and endurance, speed and agility, the object is never to injure an opponent. Injuries that do occur among youngsters include a pulled elbow, where the head of the radius pops out of alignment. It can be clicked back into place by a qualified person. Because players often resist throws with the fist clenched, "judo elbow" is produced, with a pain on both sides of the joint, often described as a combination of **tennis** and **golf elbow**.

Apart from general twists and strains, there are disfigurements such as **cauliflower ears** and even permanently bent fingers where a player has repeatedly used a favourite technique that strains ligaments and results in joint displacement.

Shoulder injuries, from poor landings, are common and can be severe – **A/C separation, dislocation** – so should always be treated by a doctor. Back injuries are mainly facet and sacroiliac related and respond to manipulation. In tournaments where several bouts are contested, fluid balance must be maintained.

Karate
See: Martial arts.

Kayaking
See: Canoeing.

Netball
See: Basketball.

Racquetball
See: Squash.

Rowing

Traditionally, a number of rowing injuries came from land-based training, but nowadays the rowing ergometer (rowing machine) enables rowers to train on dry land while mimicking rowing. As this is a power sport, overload and back injuries (disc displacements) are common from training too hard, often in poor positions. Make certain your weight lifting technique is correct and only compete against yourself – not the person working out next to you. If you do get knee tracking problems, then this can be corrected by placing a backstop on the slide at a distance that ensures that the knees straighten. The slide must hit the backstop with each stroke.

In the boat, **upper back pain** is often a facet joint pain but may be felt in the ribs or the chest. Stress fractures of the ribs are not unknown, so a positive rib spring or a point tenderness on a rib might well need a bone scan. The cause of high back pain is overreaching on the stroke or sudden loss of balance in the boat when catching the water. Manipulate early.

Mid-back pain can also be caused by overreaching producing a hunched middle-back position. Ensure neutral back position through the stroke. Take any weight training slowly, ensuring correct technique.

The gripping and twisting action of rowing produces **paddler's wrist** (see: Canoeing) where the long tendon and sheath of the thumb are inflamed in the wrist and forearm. Cross-frictional massage, ultrasound and an injection of cortisone may help, but surgery may be required to release constriction of the sheath. Enthusiastic beginners who try to do too much in one session may suffer this. It usually occurs in the feathering hand. Experienced rowers may flare the wrist by an alteration in the oar handle size (too small, too large), in rough weather or even if the gate is too tight.

Rugby, Union and League

In a game that involves catching and passing a ball, proper techniques must be learned to minimize finger injuries (**mallet fingers**) as well as to increase skill. Tackling and taking a tackle properly are important for both playing effectively and avoiding injury.

Hamstring problems are common amongst the backs, who have to stand around doing little, waiting for the ball. Backs should never stand still but always keep loose, moving, ready. However, proper stretching lowers the risk, especially for the explosive, short-stepping sprinters like halfbacks, who tend to have shorter hamstrings.

Forwards need to have powerful necks and backs. Special training is necessary at schoolboy level where a worrying number of paralysis injuries have been incurred in recent years. This can be due to mismatching – grading teams by age rather than size. At the highest level, rugby authorities have recognized that the front row is a specialist position and can only have a specialized player as a substitute or replacement. Incorrect scrummaging causes aches and pains, too.

In a game of physical contact, **concussion** is not uncommon. As the brain has been bruised, the player should maintain fitness but not play matches for three weeks (see: Concussion, p. 43).

When **neck pain** occurs amongst forwards, it could be caused by lack of specific strength in the neck and shoulders, or by discs that could have been moved; seek medical advice.

Back pain, when not due to bruising, is not caused by pulling a muscle during a ruck or maul but by damage to a ligament, disc or facet joint. Seek medical advice and do not play until advised. Ensure neutral position (p. 79) in the scrum.

Shoulders take the brunt of falls, often producing the **A/C joint injury**. Use a sling early on and avoid weight training with the arms until cured. Seek medical help, because in rare cases forwards may need surgery. Diving with the ball in both outstretched hands to score a try can cause shoulder dislocation, but the most common cause is the fall back tackle. Indeed those with unstable shoulders should not play in the centre or fullback. Non-union of the collarbone might allow for other sports but will not permit a tackle.

Groin strains can be dealt with using the ladder principle: Build up the sidestep gradually through the knee run (p. 138), but beware violent sidesteps that may produce **Footballer's groin**. Build into punting and kicking, looking for easy rhythm and accuracy until pain free. Then add length.

With the increased emphasis on fitness training, using weights that are too heavy for too long will produce overuse injuries. Knee overload is typical. Goal kickers may flare the injury after a long session using a heavy ball. A tackle blocking the kicking leg while punting or even a tackle which prevents completion of the knee straightening (while running) can cause **quads pull**. If **torn cartilage ligaments** are the problem, avoid using the bad knee when getting up during training sessions. Props can benefit from changing from loose to tight head (or vice versa) if the front knee is the problem, but swollen knees from anterior cruciate and cartilage are moderately frequent.

Ugly **cauliflower ears** can be prevented by using a headband and draining the blood from the ear early on.

Running
See: Track and Field Athletics.

Sailing
Whether you are out at leisure or in a competition, dehydration is a problem – even if you are surrounded by water. Take plastic bottles with plastic straws, so that you can drink while racing. The presence of water always increases the risk of hypothermia, sunburn or eye glare, so wear the appropriate gear. The leaning, bending and pulling required give the back and stomach muscles a fair workout, but in larger boats, larger loads can cause strains, so maintain correct techniques, especially maintain a neutral back position when pulling, lifting or winding. Knee ligaments can suffer when

the dinghy helmsman is forced to sit in an awkward position. Try other positions.

Silly accidents can be avoided: Know the distance between the bottom of the boom and the top of the deck or centreboard case; don't stand near coils of heavy-duty rope; keep your hands and fingers well away from winches and pulleys. Seasickness can be helped by tablets, but these make some people drowsy, so special wristbands may be the alternative. Consult doctor.

Scuba Diving
See: Swimming.

Shooting
Ear protection should be worn at all times to prevent deafness (acoustic trauma). Apart from accidents with weapons, there are few injuries in the sport. Shoulders and faces can be bruised and even cut due to "kick", which is made worse by a badly fitting gun. Avoid this by:
• Getting a gun of the correct size and shape, with correct mounting and good stock fitting. For some wrist (**De Quervain**) and **elbow injuries**, a switch to a "pistol grip" may help.
• Holding the gun more firmly. The thumb should always be curled around the stock, not left behind the top lever, which can come back and damage the thumb. When the gun is held properly, there should be 3 fingers' space between thumb and nose.

Housemaid's knee may occur in the kneeling position of 3-position rifle shooting. A padded plastic or rubber knee pad helps.

Many shooters require drugs for medical conditions such as heart trouble or high blood pressure. Some drugs, such as beta blockers, are banned for competition, so a doctor should be consulted about changing the tablets.

Skating, Ice
Speed skating, because of its forward lean, may produce **high knee hip pain.** Training should be built up gradually, and hip strength should be maintained with squat thrusts and burpees.

In artistic or figure skating, the top performers are often injured when the huge jumps and spins attempted are not completed. At lower levels, when knee overload occurs, avoid jumps until better. Work on tracing figures and straight-line step sequence. When improving, try to alternate days for work on jumps. Tracking problems of the knee may occur if the knee is not held vertically over the foot during one-leg, bent-knee balance.

Stress fractures may occur through repeating the same jump too often in one session. The check and pick of the foot with rotation causes strain through the leg bones, especially from triple lutzes. Plan the week so that jump sessions are not too long on any one day, and if possible alternate between days with jumps and days without jumps.

Tailbone pain (coccygitis) is very painful and can be caused by repeated falling. It is more frequent among women.

Ice hockey injuries are primarily from violent physical contact. Skater's heel is often the result of wearing boots that are too tight in the heel, while **interdigital neuritis** (**Morton's foot pain**) is caused by too narrow a boot at the toes, so make sure they fit properly.

The rapid pump of legs to build up speed may produce thigh muscle strain or even pull-off fracture, while the violent checking can cause overload problems of the knees.

Skiing

Most skiers are holiday makers who do little or no physical preparation. Travellers who would worry about going to the altitude of Mexico City think nothing of exerting themselves in the mountains. No wonder dehydration and altitude sickness (nausea, dizzy spells, headaches, tiredness) are common. Take liquid – not alcohol – and allow time to adjust. As snow reflects 85 per cent of the sun's burning rays, use wraparound sunglasses and a sunscreen recommended by your doctor. When cross-country skiing, remember to take an outward course that leaves you with enough energy to get back comfortably! Replace liquids frequently. Mittens, where all the fingers are together, are warmer than gloves, and if the extremities (nose, ears, toes, fingers) go numb and red, keep moving so that the circulation has a chance to help. The head loses a lot of heat, so always wear a hat. Never go off to explore an unfamiliar mountain without a survival bag and a map of the pistes at the very least. Those skiing at the back of a group often have no idea where they are and should be made to read the route plan regularly.

Thanks to modern boot and binding design, as well as to better instruction, injuries are less frequent than they used to be. However, good stretching and preparation can minimize accidents further. Get the best ski bindings; don't have them too tight and ensure that they are properly mounted, set and oiled and freed up daily as the cold will stiffen the bindings.

Pain, numbness or pins and needles that persist over the top of the foot and the big toe can be caused by pressure of the boots on a nerve, either in the leg, at the top front of the ankle or over the forefoot. Improve the padding, loosen it or get a larger pair of boots.

Medial ligament strain, knee tracking problems and **torn cartilage ligaments** usually occur in the less able skier, who cannot parallel properly and stem turn. Holding the neutral position (p. 79) may help weight adjustment as will keeping the knees over the feet – "not knock-kneed" in the schuss position. If good skiers have knee problems, their bindings are probably too tight. Even sitting on the backs of your skis and then pulling upright has been known to "pop" the anterior cruciate ligament. Check your bindings to reduce this injury in falls. A slow fall that does not release the binding often produces a calf muscle pull.

Knee overload is flared by fast runs in the "egg" position, or when mogul running/racing. Relax on easier runs. Technique may suffer badly with knee overload, and slalom should not be undertaken until leg power is within 10 per cent of the strength of the other leg.

In cross-country skiing, **anterior compartment pain** is an overuse injury caused when the toes and forefoot are lifted toward the shinbone on the prolonged forward glide, especially on hard uphill sessions. Build up strength with toe-hold sit-ups and correct technique. **Tennis elbow** is an overuse injury caused by the action of planting the ski-pole and twisting it free for the next stride, while poling can cause **triceps strain**.

Skier's thumb occurs when the ligaments at the base of the thumb are torn by the ski-pole straps or the "diamonds" on a dry ski slope. Dry slope skiers can try mittens or even a sock over their hands as this will push out between thumb and index finger during the fall and may stop the thumb from catching in the matting. Thermoplastic thumb splints may be individually made to prevent the problem.

Soccer

Cuts, bruises and broken bones are common enough, but most injuries are in the lower limbs. **Footballer's groin** is thought to be brought on by the one-sided load of kicking. In defenders, it is flared by backing off and twisting from side to side and can be difficult to distinguish from adductor muscle strains. You can play through the early stage or rest for 9-12 months, but it may need surgery to return faster. Get an opinion from an experienced sports doctor. When fit for sprints, use the

Achilles top ladder, and at step 7 start a simultaneous kicking ladder:

1 Juggle ball.
2 Stroke ball 10 yd.
3 Chip.
4 Drive and volley.
5 Inside of foot drive.
6 Hooked kick.
7 Tackle gently.
8 Lower-level game.
9 Channelling opponents one way only.
10 Match fit.

Adductor strains are often caused by overstretching sideways or a blocked sidefoot tackle. Use the kicking ladder (above) to build back. **Quads pull** can be the result of someone blocking your leg as you straight drive or volley the ball. However, knee overload is usually caused in training rather than match play, when a long session of quadriceps work plus hard kicking, especially with a heavy ball, flares the injury. Alter the training and reduce quads strength training.

The twisting strains of ball control are particularly severe on the knee and **torn cartilage** or **cartilage ligaments** can result. Avoid close dribbling in training, especially when carrying the ball with the injured leg. Checking the ball with the outside of the foot can cause trouble. Defenders should channel attackers so that you turn on your good side (or even switch sides of the field to make this easier) and tell covering team-mates which way you will channel. In training, do not do bunny hops and avoid using the bad leg when getting up from the ground.

Front of ankle joint strain occurs after repeated kicking of a heavy ball or after a drive is blocked. Use stirrup strapping (p. 113) on both sides of the ankle to try to prevent the foot being forced down when driving the ball. Build up through chip and side foot to drive and volley in practice. Jumper's ankle can occur, too, if a blocked drive kick forces the heelbone onto the back of the shin. It is probably safe to play, but the injury will not settle until treated medically. **Footballer's ankle** from repeated knocks and sprains is usually sore at rest, but feels better on the move.

Softball

See: Baseball.

Squash/Racquetball

These are classic games for getting fit, but always play within the boundaries of your own fitness because it is easy to overdo it. It is not "soft" to wear proper eye protection as the ball fits the eye socket neatly, which can be dangerous. Always call lets or penalty points rather than hit the ball if you think you are likely to hit your opponent. The hard floors can produce blisters and **black nail**, and in hot climates, fluid intake is important. Shoulder injuries are common.

A/C joint pain is usually no trouble unless you play a lot of overheads, so avoid smashes and take off the back wall – unless it's a vital match! Using a flying elbow instead of rotating properly may cause trouble on the forehand, especially **shoulder impingement** from the **subacromial bursa**, but in severe cases,

the backhand may hurt. Seek medical advice. If you suffer from **painful arc** (caused by squash) you should check with a coach as your technique needs correcting. Hitting volley boasts or cutting forehand while hitting off the racquet foot (i.e. front on) may flare biceps tendon.

Squash player's finger is caused by using a closed grip with the index finger extended too far down the shaft and holding too tightly, causing pain in the bulky muscle on the back of the hand between thumb and index finger. Use the 3rd, 4th and 5th fingers to grip. Knee overload may cause trouble over the knee on the racquet-hand side.

Pronator terres syndrome is caused by faulty technique, where the forehand is played with the racquet-hand below the wrist. Injury occurs trying to angle the shot straight to the front wall on forehand retrieve instead of hitting the boast. Correct the fault.

Outer strap tendon pains may be induced by rolling over the outer side of the foot when playing backhand. Alter your technique and use a lateral wedge, ankle support or stirrup strapping.

Tennis elbow/squash elbow is caused by either a lack of forearm strength and/or faulty technique. On the forehand using a closed grip, the index finger is forced too far along the handle and there is a tendency to drop the racquet head and play an arm shot with the elbow flying and lack of upper body rotation. In a faulty backhand, the racquet head drops and the elbow leads the racquet into a shot. Correct your technique and check that your grip is not held tightly by thumb and forefinger. Try a thicker handle and grip with the 3rd, 4th and 5th fingers. Use the squash ladder to get back to fitness. **Olecranon fossa impingement** is caused by a backhand shot hit with a straight elbow.

Surfing
See: Swimming.

Swimming/Scuba diving/Surfing/Water polo

Swimming is regarded as the ideal form of exercise because it is so injury-free. However, everyone should know that it is dangerous to swim soon after a meal as stomach cramp is possible. Chlorine in pools, if too strong, can bleach hair and sting the eyes and may stimulate asthma in the sensitive, while verruca warts can be caught from the damp floors of public poolsides. If you have them, wear rubber swimsocks to be fair to others. Do not poke at blocked up ears, even with cotton buds. This can scratch the surface, causing chronic infection.

Physical problems only really emerge when swimmers become competitive, training for 30 miles (50 km.) a week combined with heavy dry land training. The result is overuse injuries such as swimmer's shoulder – **painful arc, shoulder impingement, subacromial bursa.**

Crawler's compression is caused by applying shoulder power before completion of arm recovery. This "striking too soon" may cause swimmer's shoulder.

In the breaststroke, there can be knee ligament problems which can be corrected by reducing the width of the leg kick to the width of the shoulders and increasing the backward kick, wedge kick rather than frog kick. Freestyle and butterfly can produce back, patella and ligament problems, which are corrected by improving the quality of the stroke as well as by reducing distance in training. For extreme butterfly problems, especially stress fracture of the spine **(bowler's back)**, change the stroke and practise backstroke for a while, before building up through freestyle and then returning to butterfly.

Scuba diving has its inherent safety problems, which must never be treated lightly. The "bends" are a decompression sickness where gas forms bubbles in the bloodstream; "rapture of the depths" is nitrogen narcosis; burst lungs are the result of an air embolism. Stick to the scuba diving safety drill all the time.

Surfing is dangerous thanks to the combination of fast-moving water and heavy boards that can knock a swimmer senseless. However, there are two or three afflictions peculiar to the sport:
• Wax rash is caused by lying on the board, so wear a T-shirt. The T-shirt also prevents sunburn.
• Surfer's foot is a painful growth at the head of the first metatarsal bone produced when the body's weight is over the instep of one foot when propelling the board out to sea.
• Wetsuit rub is cured by applying petroleum jelly to the sore part and checking that the suit fits properly.

Water polo is a tough sport, but apart from the results of physical contact, the shoulders can suffer stiffness due to overuse. Impingement from throwing is often the cause; work on throwing technique might well help.

Tennis

Most recreational players use a standard grip and single backhand, while top amateurs and professionals are switching to a Western or Semi-Western grip. The two styles produce different injuries when not properly executed. Consult a coach on technique.

The sport's most famous ailment is **tennis elbow**, which can be caused either by lack of forearm strength or by a technical fault, using the standard grip. Sometimes an awkward bounce can flare the injury, too. If you play your forehand with a closed grip and hit the ball with an open stance, you will tend to have an "arm only" swing without shoulder rotation. The racquet head is too low, and the elbow is put under stress. Correct your technique.

By contrast, the Western grip allows for this shot. Players using the two-handed backhand rarely suffer from tennis elbow. Using the single-handed backhand, the sloppy backhand punch is common, with the ball pushed with the elbow. The elbow should be tucked in, pointing towards the ground, not the net. When the racquet head is below wrist level and the high wrist leads into the shot, the power is generated by the wrist. These muscles, however, start at the elbow, and it is there that they suffer. Correct your technique. It may be worth trying a thicker racquet grip with a

lighter-weight head and less taut stringing. Use the Tennis ladder plan to regain fitness.

Radiohumeral joint/Triceps strain can be the result of tension during a match, which often makes you grip your racquet more tightly with thumb and index finger. This prevents the wrist from releasing, especially in topspin service, causing a snapping effect at the elbow, which may also flare the triceps. Relax this thumb/index finger pressure, cut down the speed and jerk of your service, ensure the ball is being thrown in front and hit through the shot. The backhand grip for service encourages this snap into extension and can flare the radio humeral joint. Consult a coach.

Pronator terres syndrome is usually caused when retrieving a forehand shot that is nearly past you, so the racquet head is dropped below the wrist; more of a hurried shot than a technical fault. More likely with the Semi-Western or extreme Western grip are impingement injuries of the bones in the wrist. Sometimes the end of the racquet handle will dig into the butt of the hand and cause **ulnar nerve compression** or **pisiform strain**. Hold the handle shorter.

With all the running involved (and good footwork is essential), **arthritis** or **rigid toe** injury in the big toe may occur. When the service action levers across the big toe of the back foot, this can flare the big toe joint. Try a jump serve to avoid this.

The repetitive serve action will always reflare a damaged **A/C joint**, which will require rest and treatment. However, bad technique such as being front on at the serve may strain the shoulder muscles, and power generated at the shoulder may produce **subdeltoid bursa, rotator cuff, shoulder impingement**. Try taking the tennis racquet back high over the shoulder into the hitting position – rather than low and backward and then throwing the ball up to hit. Tennis is a game for all ages, but shoulder problems due to alteration in circulation occur more frequently in the older person producing frozen shoulder. Ground strokes can usually be improved while the shoulder is being treated; remember that leg and knee injuries should not prevent you from practising strokes against a tennis-training machine.

Track and Field Athletics

More time is spent training than competing. Most of the injuries occur in the legs and are covered earlier in the book. Some ailments are peculiar to different events. Imitating a champion's training method may not be right for your shape and size. Quantity is no substitute for quality in running events, so more miles do not necessarily mean better results. Artificial tracks are quite hard (as are roads), so train on grass when it comes to quantity. Keep your quality for the track. Track and field enthusiasts tend to be swayed by fads – diets, vitamins, even equipment. Many of these are expensive but don't improve performance.

Groin strain, adductor muscle strain and **adductor pull-off**: Sometimes caused by weak hip flexors (the psoas) doing high knee drills.

• Sprints: Delay block starts until healed, then use cruise out starts over the first week to build up adductor strength. Bend running should be built up from the outside lane. After 6 runs without pain, move in a lane. Repeat, moving inward.
• Discus: Jerky rotations can cause problems. Concentrate on footwork.
• Hurdles: Beware the complication of **footballer's groin**, especially with high hurdles.

Knee overload:

Sprints: Avoid weight training and sprint starts for quads until healed. Use rolling starts.

Long, triple jump: Rest from jumping; work on speed. Beware of bounding and step-ups. Use the Quads ladder.

Jumper's knee: Repeated minor damage to the kneecap tendon produces thickening of the tendon lining. This may require surgery. It is important that Quads and Knee ladders are followed carefully, not rushed, or the injury will recur.

Knee tracking: Correct with orthotics – but particularly work on hip strength and keeping knee over feet during gait cycle of foot.

Cartilage ligament strain:

Pole vault: If the high knee approach is over-emphasized, the lower leg may flail (or windmill) on the carry side to counterbalance upper body rotation. Check with a coach.

Medial ligament strain:

Sprints: Use a rolling start until pain free; use outer lanes for bend running.

Javelin thrower's elbow: An overuse injury thought to be caused by round-arm technique. Dangerous when occurring in growing youngsters. Seek medical advice, as a piece of bone may pull off. Takes 4-6 weeks to heal.

Hamstring pull: Sprinters should watch their change of cadence as they go from the starting body angle to the more upright, flowing angle. Pull-off fractures are fairly common among teenagers. It is possible that the damaged leg may be the stronger, suffering damage from working too hard making up for the other weaker leg. Isokinetic assessment may help.

Triple jumper's heel: Heel cups help, but avoid jumping if possible. Work on speed; use standing jumps.

Shot putter's finger: Rare. A sprain of the first 3 fingers from squeezing the shot to give a final acceleration to the putt. Rest from throwing, tape (check for legality in competition) and use laser, ultrasound and cortisone injections. Omit finger acceleration in training throws; save for competition.

Fosbury flop ankle: Pain occurs on the outer side of the ankle in high jumpers who use the flop-styled over-everted foot at plant for take off. As the foot checks for rotation, the momentum drives the bone against the central hinge, the talus. Using self-diagnosis, the foot hurts when the heel is forced sideways and outward, but does not hurt on forcing the heel inward or when pulling the toes downward and inward as with a twisted ankle. Rest will help, along with correction of the technical fault. Cortisone injections, even surgery, may be needed. Subsequent training should concentrate on heels, quads, stretching. Maintain straight-line bounding and depth jumping. Build into Fosbury rotation, straighten foot plant.

Stress fractures: Sprinters, hurdlers and jumpers are more prone to navicular stress fractures. Long-distance runners tend to have stress fractures of the shin (tibia) and low fibula area. Compartment syndromes of the calf can occur in middle- and long-distance runners. The anterior compartment hurts in runners who shuffle without much drive from the forefoot. Do not run distances that break your bones! Rest them by interspersing a heart/lung session on your pedal bike – your fitness will be the same, and your body won't fall apart! Try a varied weekly routine: Monday – long, steady bike session (the bike equivalent to running is about 2 to 2½ times the distance in the same time), Tuesday – long run, Wednesday – bike session, Thursday – short run, getting up to full racing speed, Friday – rest, Saturday – race, Sunday – race.

Joggers should ease into their sport. Running is a skill that can be taught but very rarely is. Running, however slowly, along a beach with its soft sand does the Achilles tendon no good at all for a first-time workout. Avoid running hard downhill. This is a great temptation but jars the spine, knee, etc. The camber on the road can alter the impacts going through the body and cause problems – so if you run on a cambered surface – change sides at regular intervals. To avoid running too fast, too soon, try chatting, talking to yourself or a partner.

If you can't, you are going too fast. Those with pronated feet and especially children over 7 may be helped by orthotics, which give a solid base instead of the soft collapsing foot on which to run. In spite of help from orthotics, however, some anatomies will keep breaking down because they are not made to run – look for other sports.

Trampolining
See: Diving and Trampolining.

Triathlon
See: Track and Field Athletics, Cycling, Swimming.

Volleyball
See: Basketball.

Water polo
See: Swimming.

Water skiing
Travelling at speed with the possibility of crashing will always mean that injuries are not far away. Water is much harder than you think when you hit it at speed – as is the shore if you dismount too late! Once you get to competition level, there are knee ligament problems and dislocated shoulders, which can occur in slalom, and heel spur (plantar fasciitis) which can occur as the jump ski hits the ramp – pad the ski, try dye strapping, but heel cups may not stay in place.

At lower levels, a good level of fitness is required to avoid knee and shoulder strains. Early overuse strains such as **tennis elbow** (from holding the tow handle horizontally) may be eased by turning the handle vertical, loading the biceps muscles instead of the elbow. Beginners must ensure that wetsuits protect the groin area, otherwise a high-pressure douche or enema (amusing to talk about but excruciatingly painful) can occur when water is forced up the front or back passage. Recreational skiers should always have a driver and watcher on board to avoid serious accidents from the propeller or tow rope to others in the water.

Weight lifting/Weight Training
One fitness expert considered weight training the most worrying sport that he encountered. Equipment is often readily available without qualified supervision and this, coupled with most people's competitive nature (as when two friends try to outlift one another), can cause unseen injuries, especially among youngsters. Fortunately, most gyms have competent, trained staff to advise on a personal programme: use this advice when available. Children whose bones have not fused (fully grown), should not be weight training.

Knee overload is likely when the quads muscles are overloaded. Build up weights gradually, and if the knees ache, decrease weight and concentrate on lifting technique. Build up upper body strength. Knee supports may act like an outer skeleton, spreading the load from these pressure points. Repeat training of squats and splits while injured will not allow these injuries to heal.

A dislocated elbow can occur if a

weight is lifted with too much backward component instead of vertical acceleration. Trying to hold this weight above the head, especially in the snatch, may cause dislocation. Check the pulse. Use a sling. Get medical help.

Weight trainers would do better with counterbalanced, as opposed to free, weights, so that they can sit down with the back supported (as in power gyms). Once you throw your back into a lift, it means the muscle group you are training has fatigued. If you have back problems – stop at this weight and make this the endpoint of your repetition. It is worth remembering that high loads, low repetitions give you strength; low loads, high repetitions give you stamina. To develop power, a weight needs to be moved quickly. Build up to the heaviest weight you can manage while still able to move it quickly. Most sports require that power equals speed and strength, so work weights explosively and build up weight maintaining same explosive speed for that muscle. Pectoral decks must not allow the shoulders to go too far backward, otherwise **dislocated/subluxed shoulder** can occur. Keep elbows below shoulder height to prevent **shoulder impingement.**

Dehydration can be a problem as weight lifters try to get into the lowest weight category.

Wrestling

Wrestling is one of those sports that is well supervised and well coached so there is a relatively low incidence of technical injury. Basic throwing and falling techniques are essential. Joints (shoulders, knees, ankles) suffer from the wrenches of both competition and training and must be treated appropriately. Hands and wrists are hurt from bad falls, while **cauliflower** or **wrestler's ear** is a regular problem, though school and college grapplers wear protective headgear.

Dehydration can be a problem as wrestlers try to get into the lowest weight category to maximize their strength. The problem of combining weight control (diet) with top-level fitness (per cent of body fat) is different for each individual.

6

A-Z of Medical Terms

Sports doctors, like all doctors, often use long and technical words for quite simple injuries, which can be a worry. There is no need to panic; just look up that word here. (See also: A-Z of Treatments, Chapter 2.)

Abdominals Stomach muscles

A/C joint/acromio clavicular joint Joint between collarbone and shoulder blade; forms step in shoulder if displaced.

Acromion Bony tip of shoulder; tip of shoulder blade.

Aerobics Continuous exercise at three-quarter speed and below; raises pulse rate to improve heart and lung function and strengthen muscles for greater stamina.

Amenorrhoea Absence of periods. (See p. 21).

Amino acids Building blocks for protein, which may be of benefit in overtraining syndrome and sprint work. Some have produced bad reactions.

Anaemia Insufficient red cells in blood. Small measured variations do not alter athletic performance. May have number of causes, but check with doctor, especially if periods heavy.

Anaerobic Muscle exercise without oxygen; only lasts short time, with high pulse rate, e.g., explosive events like sprinting, weight lifting.

Anterior Front.

Arthritis Greek for inflammation of the joint. Surface of joint wears, resulting in pain. Wear-and-tear of cartilage and bone of joint or disease such as rheumatoid or psoriatic arthritis or Lyme disease may contribute to condition.

Arthrogram X-ray technique for joints using air and/or dye injected into joint, to reveal torn cartilage. Less common since advent of magnetic resonance imaging (MRI).

Arthroscope Modern technique using fibre optics to probe complex joints such as knee, shoulder, ankle and wrist to track down injury and even operate. Sort of telescope that can look into joint. Arthroscopy is name of operation.

Asthma Constriction of tubes to lungs so breathing becomes difficult. (See: Some sensible tips, p. 14.)

Biceps Bulging muscle on front of upper arm, the "Popeye muscle", used to bend elbow.

Biceps femoris One of hamstring muscles.

Bone scan Uses radioactive dye (equivalent of 1 x-ray) to scan for stress fractures, etc.

Bursa Sac of fluid that cushions or

greases movement of skin, muscles, tendons or ligaments across hard area and so stops them from fraying (like string rubbing over brick). When inflamed, condition is known as bursitis.

Calcaneum Heel bone.

Capsule Lining linking bone to bone; contains lubricating fluid for joint. See: Ligament.

Cardiovascular To do with heart and circulation. In sporting terms, implies ability to move oxygen from lungs to muscles and to get rid of carbon dioxide, body's exhaust fumes.

Cartilage Smooth, slippery substance that prevents two ends of bones from grating. Cartilage may become torn. Knee has extra shock absorbers between the cartilage-covered bones, known as the cartilage or meniscus. Complete removal leads to arthritis, so surgeons repair a.tear or try to remove as little of the meniscus as possible.

Chondromalacia Roughening of slippery cartilage surface. Best known is chondromalacia patellae, or roughening of underside of kneecap.

Clavicle Collarbone.

Closed chain exercises Physiotherapy term for exercising muscles.

Concentric Muscle working as it shortens.

Congenital From birth, or within the genes.

Conjoined tendon Tendon of abdominal muscles that attaches to front of pelvis; weakness gives footballer's groin or hernia.

Contrast baths Using heat followed by cold to increase blood flow.

Contusion Bruise.

Costal To do with ribs.

CT scan Computer takes x-ray pictures of slices of body to make a series of pictures. Very good for checking bones.

Crepitus Grating feeling over damaged joint or tendon.

Cross-frictional massage Technique of rubbing, using small movements but firm pressure across line of muscle or tendon growth. Thought to break down scar tissue and realign fibres.

Deep friction massage Uses firm pressure to get at deeper tissues.

Deltoids Muscles at top of arm, just below shoulder, which lift from about 20 degrees at the side up to 160 degrees.

Dorsiflex Bending foot and ankle upward.

Eccentric Muscle working as it lengthens.

Effluage Massage technique to remove swelling.

EKG/ECG (Electrocardiogram)
Recording of heart's electrical activity.

EMG (Electromyograph) Checks how well nerve muscle complex is working.

Exercise cardiogram
EKG/electrocardiogram performed during exercise.

Extension Straightening/over-straightening joint.

Facet joint Joints of spine joining vertebrae together.

Fast twitch fibre See: White fibre.

Femur Big thighbone in upper leg.

Fibula Smaller bone on outside of lower leg. Lower end forms outer anklebone.

Flexion Opposite of extension, i.e. bending joint.

Fracture Broken bone.

Gait Running or walking style.

Gastrocnemius Part of calf muscle.

Hamstring Muscle at back of thigh that bends knee.

Haematoma Pocket of congealed blood, bigger and more serious than bruise.

Often causes a raised lump as blood vessels are broken and bleed.

Humerus Bone of upper arm.

Impingement Banging together of two surfaces not normally in contact. Implies movements greater than normal range, e.g., gymnasts arching backward.

Inflammation Damage from overuse, wear and tear, or disease; not from outside source.

Interferential Electrical machine to heat muscles and joints. Can also stimulate muscles and control pain.

Isokinetic exercises Isokinetic means same energy. Muscles vary in power in different positions, following principle of leverage. Sprinters start in crouch because more power is released from that position. Isokinetic machines are complex, costly and may help diagnosis and indicate type of training.

Isometric exercises Isometric means same length. Two equal forces working against each other produce no movement. Used to test muscle and tendon pain, also to build strength that is angle specific, i.e. only in position of exercise, not all positions.

Isotonic drinks Isotonic is a marketing, not a medical term. In this sense it refers to fluids that replace water and sweat. If energy needed as well, special sugars may be added.

Isotonic exercises For strength-building as in weight lifting or with now-popular "variable resistance" machines in gymnasiums and health clubs. Idea is to shorten and lengthen muscles with same weight.

Laceration Cut.

Lactic acid Waste product of muscle energy. As this builds up, muscles cease to work. Sprint/endurance exercises build lactic acid faster, hence sudden loss of leg strength at end of 440 yd. (400 m.). See: OBLA.

Laser Used for both surgery and for treatment.
• Surgical laser used like a knife, but actually vaporizes tissue.
• Therapeutic laser uses different wavelength of light to surgical laser. Similar to ultrasound in its effect. Often less effective after four treatments.

Lateral Outer side of body.

Ligament Area strengthening joints, linking bone to bone, e.g., forearm to upper arm.

Loose body Free fragment of bone or cartilage floating inside joint.

Medial Inner side of body.

Metacarpals Five bones of hand, just before fingers. One end forms the knuckles.

Metatarsals Five bones of foot, just before toes.

Microwave Not oven, but electrical equipment to heat deep tissues.

MRI or Magnetic resonance imaging. Body scan for bone, disc, brain and soft tissue.

NSAIDs Non-steroidal anti-inflammatory drugs. Best known is aspirin; made as creams or gels as well. Many of these available at drugstore.

OBLA Stands for: Onset Blood Lactic Acid, during exercise. Usually referred to by level, such as OBLA 2 or OBLA 4. Yet another fitness measurement.

Oligomenorrhoea Very light periods (see p. 21).

Open chain exercises Physiotherapy term for exercising muscles.

Osteochondritis Damage through cartilage and bone.

Osteoporosis Disease in which bones become brittle, a characteristic of old age. Physical activity increases strength of bones. Absence of menstrual periods decreases bone strength. Hormone replacement therapy (HRT) may prevent fractures.

Patella Kneecap.

Pectorals Chest muscles, beneath breast leading up to shoulder.

Plantarflex Bending foot and ankle downward.

Prolotherapy Sugar injections into ligaments to strengthen them.

Quads/Quadriceps Muscles of thigh that straighten knee.

Radius Forearm bone on thumb side.

Red fibre Part of muscle that maintains slower, weaker and longer-lasting work. Also known as slow twitch fibre.

Referred pain Pain felt in undamaged area of body away from actual injury. Conceals real source of injury.

Resting pulse Pulse taken first thing in morning before getting out of bed.

Rotator cuff Group of deep muscles that fix and control the shoulder, holding the humerus into the scapula.

Sacroiliac joint Two joints in pelvis at back.

Scapula Shoulder blade.

Sesamoid bone Lies within and adds strength to tendons as they cover bony point; best known is kneecap.

Short leg Phrase used by osteopaths to explain rotation in pelvis; not one leg shorter than the other. True short leg can only be diagnosed by x-ray. Most people tolerate 1 in. (1-2 cm.) difference in leg length without problem. Some may require orthotics.

Shortwave diathermy Deep heat treatment on joints. See: Interferential, Microwave.

Slow twitch fibre See: Red fibre.

Soleus Calf muscle.

SPECT scan Single Photon Emission Computerized Tomography. Extremely sensitive bone scan.

Sprain Damage to ligament or lining of joint.

Sternum Breastbone.

Steroids Group of chemicals produced in body.
• Anabolic steroids occur naturally and help to build muscles but are banned when tablets or injections are used to enhance performance.
• Catabolic steroids such as cortisone help to break down or control inflammation. Again banned when given externally under certain circumstances.

Strain Damage to muscle or tendon.

Strap muscles Balance muscles of feet.

Stress fracture Break in bone caused by continual repetition of same movement.

Synovial fluid Lubricating fluid for joints and tendons, produced in synovium, or inner lining of joint. Synovitis is damage to synovium.

Talus Foot bone that hinges in between two anklebones.

Tendon Joins muscle to bone. Tendons are unable to contract and relax; may be very long, as on back of hand. Tendinitis is damage to tendon.

Tenosynovitis Inflammation of both tendon and sheath surrounding it.

Tibia Larger of two bones in lower leg/shinbone.

Trauma Damage caused by blow or outside source.

Triceps Muscles in upper arm that extend elbow.

Ulna One of two bones in forearm; forms point of elbow and lies on little finger side.

White fibre Part of muscle that produces fast, strong, but not long-lasting work; builds muscle bulk. Also known as fast twitch fibre.

Xyphisternum Stomach end of breastbone; made of cartilage.

INDEX

Page numbers in **bold** indicate main references; those in *italic* indicate rehabilitation ladders.